Screenformation

D1524108

Robert Rose-Coutré

First Edition
First printing April 2018
ISBN (print book): 978-0-9973250-2-7
ISBN (e-book): 978-0-9973250-3-4
Library of Congress Control Number (LCCN): 2018900932

Cover Design by Robert Rose-Coutré and CreateSpace

Printed in the United States of America

West Chester, Pennsylvania
Rose-Coutré Publishing
2018

Table of Contents

Dedication

This book is dedicated to my wife, Mitra Rose-Coutré

Acknowledgement

I would like to acknowledge Mitra Rose-Coutré for her invaluable editorial advice.

PART I:
Brain Dysfunction

Screenformation tells the story of forty years of scientific studies showing the harmful effects of passive screentime. It provides a rich variety of published findings that prove screentime damages mental functioning, mental health, emotional development, and physical health. The book also confirms the connection between the omnipresence of screens and a dysfunctional society. It shows how first TV, then video, then passive screentime on any device, undermined the health of individuals and communities.

The first half of the book focuses on the ways screentime damages people and takes the joy out of life. It pinpoints exactly how our existence has been compromised. Just when all seems lost, the second half of the book focuses on remedies. It shines a light on our strengths, which can lead us to a richer life.

The book is firmly substantiated by hard biological science, strong psychological research, many academic studies, and expert commentary. The published evidence is overwhelming. This book brings it all together.

CHAPTER 1: WEAKENING OF BRAIN ACTIVITY

The Alpha Wave State Makes Us "Accept" Information

Based on a groundbreaking "Alpha Wave" study by Dr. Herbert E. Krugman, and others since then, the screen changes the brain by making it suggestible. Our awake state involves Beta waves. Beta waves are fast active-thinking waves, "beta waves are associated with alertness, activity." Conversely, Alpha waves are slow and are not associated with being alert. As Krugman notes, "Alpha waves are not simply slow Beta waves; they are a new parameter." Screen viewing switches the brain from Beta to Alpha waves, which are associated with hypnotism. In his Brain Wave article, Krugman explains how screen information differs from print. The reading response is "active and composed primarily of fast brain waves, whereas the response to television might be understood as passive and composed primarily of slow brain waves." Perhaps the most profound finding in the brain-wave-shift discovery was that the brain switches from active-thinking Beta Waves to passive non-thinking Alpha Waves in less than a minute from the start of viewing, and it makes no difference what's on—the screen itself causes the switch to passivity.[1]

Suggestibility makes us easier to manipulate, so we easily conform to the simulation of reality presented on the screen. That fact alone undermines brain function. An abundance of subsequent biological and psychological research has shown that screentime causes mental deterioration, altered perception of reality, and other types of damage in addition to suggestibility.[2]

Americans have an average of 189 channels on TV. On laptops, tablets, and smartphones, we are estimated to consume the equivalent of nine DVDs-worth of data per day, per person.[3] We watch TV approximately 30 hours a week.[4] We spend most of the rest of our time with smartphones, tablets, and laptops, which are also used for passive video viewing. "Young people now spend more time with media than they do in school—it is the leading activity for children and teenagers other than sleeping."[5] As a result, we spend most of every day in a passive Alpha Wave state of suggestibility. This shift to almost constant passivity and suggestibility is a new fact of our existence. The shift diminishes human variation and increases our conformity and uniformity (i.e., erodes individuality).

Alpha Waves and Critical Processing

Before the mind can analyze news and information successfully, it must be in an active state. Then it can draw comparisons and relations with sustained comprehension.

Reading or talking to another person activates the region of the brain that prepares us to logically process information and critically evaluate it. The mind is already "in gear" as it encounters arguments and concepts in a book or in a conversation.[6]

Reading and talking ignite brain cells so they can process information, but watching TV or video does the opposite. In other experiments tracking brainwaves while subjects watched TV, "The EEG studies similarly show less mental stimulation, as measured by alpha brainwave production, during viewing than during reading."[7]

Television puts the brain into a physiologically passive condition, which means we cannot critically process video-format information as reliably as reading the same information. That means we accept whatever we see "as fact" without realizing it. Our brain is not prepared to process anything competently.[8]

The screen shapes our minds to be vulnerable and receptive to simplistic screen-information, including *mis*information. Video-induced Alpha Waves make us accept bad information while making us less competent to intelligently evaluate any information.[9] With impaired logical processing, our hypnotic state renders us defenseless against manipulation.

We cannot feel the Beta-Alpha "switch" happening while we are watching screens. That lack of awareness makes us more easily influenced. We think we are processing information just fine, but in fact we are accepting information without processing it.

TV biologically prevents people from thinking for themselves. A screen-informed mind is not an informed mind. It is merely reshaped and populated by screenformation. The decision to rely on TV for information is a poor decision. It illustrates the poor judgment brought about by watching TV.

Secondhand Television

The Alpha wave state is bad for children even when they are not directly watching the screen. "Casual exposure (to TV) can harm their language development, making it harder for them to cope when they go to school ... Children are as vulnerable to the effects of 'passive TV' as they are to secondhand smoking, according to experts ... as well as discouraging the amount of screen-time to which youngsters are exposed, it cautioned against adults watching television with them nearby. It said parents needed to understand that 'their own media use can have a negative effect on children'. ... the data should serve as a 'wake up call' to parents. The American Academy of Pediatrics has included warnings about 'secondhand television' in its guidelines for children aged under two."[10]

"The risk of television delaying learning in infants is so great that the American Academy of Pediatrics recommends that babies under the age of 2 be banned from watching altogether."[11]

The Muscle Metaphor

Like a muscle, the mind needs exercise to get stronger. As a result of mental exercise, we become smarter. As *Emotional Intelligence 2.0* author and clinical psychologist Travis Bradberry notes, "your brain grows new connections much as your biceps might swell if you started curling heavy weights several times a week. The change is gradual and the weight becomes easier and easier to lift the longer you stick to your routine ... the brain cells develop new connections to speed the efficiency of thought...."[12]

By failing to exercise brain cells, they weaken and don't function as well. Screentime is not brain-exercise, it's brain-massage. Screen-stimulation acts like a delicious massage to the brain. The brain weakens like a muscle that is pleasantly massaged, but never exercised. Without exercise, the massaged mind feels good, while getting flabby. A multitude of studies and research have established the fact that passive screentime atrophies the mind. We know that screentime robs the mind of energy, thinking, problem-solving skills, logic, empathy, creativity, mental health, and emotional development.[13]

Replacing mental exercise with mental massage, people become less able to "self-stimulate" their own brains, or initiate their own mental activity, the way humans did from the beginning of human history until the mid 1900s. As the passive video experience effortlessly stimulates brain cells, so the ability to initiate one's own brain-cell activity is put to sleep, deteriorated like an atrophied muscle.[14]

Development Depends on Practice

Children are the most vulnerable to damage from the loss of mental exercise. Noted in the *Scientific Learning* article "This is Your Child's Brain on TV": "Children require face-to-face contact from caretakers who provide verbal and non-verbal clues to kids that television—no matter how kid-friendly—cannot … Since brain circuits organize and reorganize themselves in response to an infant's interactions with his or her environment, exposing babies to a variety of positive experiences (such as talking, cuddling, reading, singing, and playing in different environments) not only helps tune babies in to the language of their culture, but it also builds a foundation for developing the attention, cognition, memory, social-emotional, language and literacy, and sensory and motor skills that will help them reach their potential later on." The important takeaway here is that screentime cannot replace this foundational real-world development.[15]

For all ages, especially for younger children:
- "Watching television interrupts activities that promote cognitive and social development.

- TV can be to blame for "students who have trouble finding creative ways to solve problems, difficulty reading and seem delayed in understanding socially acceptable behavior.
- "Television causes problems because kids who watch excessively are NOT doing other things that we know will help them become academically successful.
- "TV viewing replaces reading, doing homework, pursuing hobbies and getting enough sleep. It displaces creative activities, discourages exercise, creates demand for material goods and increases aggressive behavior in some children.
- "Watching television is a passive activity, a one-way street, points out an expert on child brain development and television viewing. Television displaces other important activities that promote cognitive and social development"[16]

Screens pacify children while lowering brain function and reducing potential.

"Watching more TV in childhood increases the chances of dropping out of school and decreased chances of getting a college degree, even after controlling for confounding [socio-economic, etc.] factors ... Children who watch too much television are likely to:

- "Forego fantasy play, which is critical to brain development because it helps kids understand symbolism, the foundation of reading.
- "Fail to question and develop alternative understanding and explanations which leads to creative problem-solving.
- "Develop weaker language skills.
- "Have a diminished 'EQ,' or emotional quotient, which is critical to the development of social skills and understanding that actions have consequences. Children with compromised EQ fail to learn how to vary their responses to social experiences."[17]

Verbal Decline

Children watching TV suffer severe declines in vocabulary, which damages their ability to think. Their verbal skills are less developed than they would have been if they had not watched TV. As a variety of studies have shown, people, especially children, learn words by interacting verbally with other humans, and by watching and listening to parents in real conversations.[18] TV cannot imitate it, replace it, or even supplement it. TV can only undermine it.

To fully learn words and concepts, we have to experience the moment when words are used in real life, in relation to real people and things in a three-dimensional-world context. TV experience is not a real-world experience. If we don't experience real-world context, we don't learn as well.[19]

With real-life interaction, as with reading, the brain is activated and able to learn. The effect of TV is to turn off the learning process.

The American Academy of Pediatrics warns parents, "It may be tempting to put your infant or toddler in front of the television, especially to watch shows created just for children under age two. But the American Academy of Pediatrics says: Don't do it!"[20]

Good and Bad Comparisons

People have always been different—some better some worse— in every skill. But comparing self with others is disingenuous because it dodges the important comparison. The important comparison is self "as is" versus self "as could be."

Columbia University Professor of Psychology E. Tory Higgins explains that recognizing this discrepancy—"actual self" versus "can be" self—is referred to as self-discrepancy—"i.e., I am *not* fulfilling my potential."[21] It is known to be associated with depression: "What's wrong with me? I know I can be what I would like to be but I am not doing it."[22] It goes hand-in-hand with related sentiments about screen-viewing behaviors: "I don't want to watch as much as I do, but I can't help it."[23]

But recognizing the discrepancy between the "as is" actual self and the "as could be" or "I can be" self, is an essential step towards deciding to close the gap. Facing failed potential, the "dissatisfaction … may motivate someone to try harder. (e.g., '…Why am I so lazy? I know I can do better. I've got to try harder!')."[24]

Passive video time makes our "as is" actual self *lower functioning* than our "as could be" self. It diminishes inherited potential, regardless of how one compares with others. Over time, lower functioning manifests itself as less achievement.

Let's look at John Smith, for example:

- John Smith$_1$ grew up with an average amount of passive screentime with TV, laptop and smartphone. But he still feels he is very smart. He still knows a lot, he learns easily, and he is successful.

- John Smith$_2$ is the "as could be" or "as can be" John Smith, if only John Smith had less of a screen-centered upbringing. He is the "could be" more accomplished version, which makes the actual John Smith$_1$ look mediocre by comparison. Unfortunately, John Smith$_2$ will never exist, because John Smith's formative years were filled with screentime, and he remains in denial, refusing to address this discrepancy.

In effect, John Smith$_1$ chooses to remain John Smith$_1$. It is a lazy choice. Self-satisfied laziness is the worst possible outcome. Passive video entertainment leaves us with the second-rate version, the "as is" John Smith$_1$. Being naturally smarter that other people lulls John Smith$_1$ into the trap of self-satisfied complacency, because it's a comfortable ego boost without effort. It makes denial of the harmful effects of screentime easier.

He will never know that he was born with much more, so he will never strive to achieve more. He will never become what he could've been. As *The Motivation Myth* author Jeff Haden aptly states on the topic of this type of regret, "Sure, the work is hard. Sure, the work is painful—but it's significantly less painful than thinking back on what will never be."[25] John Smith$_2$ dies on the vine.

A better outcome is to face the discrepancy, deal with the disappointing truth, and try harder! The old saying is true: "It's not about being better than someone else, it's about being better than you were the day before."

Dysfunction became Mainstream

The loss of human abilities that we have already highlighted, has been largely uncommented in the mainstream, for two reasons. First, the change happened gradually over several generations, and became the only reality we know. Second, the change happened to everyone, which makes it less noticeable. It's like a dialect: if everyone speaks the same dialect, no one thinks it's a dialect. It's just the normal way to talk. There is no more dialect, no more differentiation, no more diversity of abilities. Everyone is the same, deteriorating in unison. Without anything to contrast against, we think our loss of abilities is just the normal way.

Each generation experiences increased frustrations, decreased initiative, devalued achievement, and lack of satisfaction. These are attributed to all kinds of things other than too much passive screentime. We keep staring at the problem under the numbing influence of Alpha Waves. We submit to its weakening effects, without grasping the root cause of our decline.

We used to build better opportunities for future generations, but we have changed that pattern. Because of our video culture, we are losing the love of learning, development of skills, willingness to struggle, and values of hard work and responsibility. Instead, we associate with lowest common denominators such as Reality Television for our standards of behavior. Digital networks become our closest personal connections.[26]

TV culture degraded the health and strength of our society, and dysfunctionality was gradually accepted as mainstream. "What television is best at doing is transforming us into passive viewers disinclined to involve ourselves with improving the political, social and economic conditions in which we live."[27]

TV Makes Us Stupid

As a recent article title says, "Watching lots of TV 'makes you stupid.'" The study piles on more evidence of what we should already know by now.

- "The study found people who watch the most TV are twice as likely to have poor mental functioning.
- "Watching TV for hours impairs your mental ability, according to study.
- "It is one of the first studies to demonstrate that watching too much TV encourages cognitive aging, even before middle age."[28]

"Several previous studies have found lower verbal IQ and increased aggressiveness in proportion to the amount of television children watch. This new research uncovers the biological mechanism for these changes in behavior and *drop in intelligence*."[29] The key here is the mathematical certainty: as hours of watching TV goes up, intelligence goes down.

The Dunning-Kruger Effect

As brain function lowers, ability to judge our own competence also decreases. As the Dunning-Kruger Effect proved, the less we can logically process information, the more we grossly overestimate our ability to logically process information.[30]

The spiraling descent of competence gains momentum: lower brain function, higher confidence in brain function; worse decision making, greater certainty of good decision making. The Dunning-Kruger Effect—the collapse of accurate self-appraisal—spreads like an intelligence-cancer. We become less smart with every hour, and more convinced that we are smarter than ever.

As David Dunning comments about his Dunning-Kruger experiments, "A whole battery of studies conducted by myself and others have confirmed that people who don't know much about a given set of cognitive, technical, or social skills tend to grossly overestimate their prowess and performance, whether it's grammar, emotional intelligence, logical reasoning, firearm care and safety, debating, or financial knowledge. College students who hand in exams that will earn them Ds and Fs tend to think their efforts will be worthy of far higher grades; [they] overestimate their competence by a long shot." He highlights the irony: "In many cases, incompetence does not leave people disoriented, perplexed, or cautious. Instead, the incompetent are often blessed with an inappropriate confidence, buoyed by something that feels to them like knowledge."[31]

Our Illusion of Knowledge

As a nation we fall further into the illusion of knowledge every decade. "A 2011 University of Chicago study found that America's college graduates 'failed to make significant gains in critical thinking and complex reasoning during their four years of college,' but more worrisome, they 'also failed to develop dispositions associated with civic engagement.' … they were less interested in applying what little they might have learned to their responsibilities as citizens." Children and younger people are especially susceptible to the tendency to read uncritically when reading on the Internet. The University College of London (UCL) study found that they typically skim and are not "evaluating information, either for relevance, accuracy or authority. … Internet users tend to … believe whichever results of a search come up first in the rankings, mostly without regard to the origins of those results." Increasingly, people believe what they see, without regard for the source, as long as it has high search ranking. Clever search-engine optimization (SEO) now trumps knowledge and truth in the minds of people "reading" on the Internet. The UCL study authors concluded that society is "dumbing down." But it gets worse. Experimental psychologists at Yale found that "'people who search for information on the Web emerge from the process with an inflated sense of how much they know' … This is a kind of electronic version of the Dunning-Kruger Effect, in which the least competent people surfing the web are the least likely to realize that they're not learning anything."[32]

The power of "mindless confidence" on a topic should not be underestimated. Even faced with hard evidence that they are incorrect, people with the illusion of knowledge simply "doubledown" on their false assumptions. People respond to truth by holding tighter to falsehood despite clear indications that they're wrong. This is the increasingly common "backfire effect" when trying to inform someone of something they don't want to know.[33]

Embracing falsehood to protect our feelings is no respecter of political orientation. As recent studies make abundantly clear, "when exposed to scientific research that challenged their views, both liberals and conservatives reacted by doubting the science, rather than themselves." Increasingly people will cling to a comfortable sense of rightness and reject the evidence.[34] We will explore this phenomenon in more detail later in the "Confirmation Bias" section.

Our society is fast becoming a prototype Dunning-Kruger experiment, where knowledge is shallow or nonexistent, while our confidence in our rightness is off-the-charts more exaggerated than ever in history. We are raising our children to make every next generation worse than the last. We think we are preparing our children for "today's technological society" by giving them more Internet time in schools and at home. We indulge them with more passive screentime than ever before. The combined effect of video, social media, and Internet "reading" results in generations of ill-equipped young men and women facing a global marketplace that will, in best case, make them suffer and struggle to get up to speed in the employment market, or worst case, crush their hopes and ruin their lives. Prisons and drug rehabs are full of them.

Productivity Decline

Passive video entertainment gave us the deadly cycle of short attention spans, weaker concentration, and less initiative. The result is the collapse of productivity from an increasingly screen-damaged employment pool.

While US workers put in long hours, we are far from the most productive. "Workers in the US put in more hours than nearly everyone but Koreans" But..."Are Americans the world's most productive employees? Not even close, according to recent research" (based on ratio of GDP to hours worked).[35] Over time, employers and employees alike begin to expect the appearance of work (long hours), but not the substance of work (productivity).

12

The American phenomenon of "presenteeism" is that "employees are expected to be at their desks not because there's so much work to be done, but simply to show their dedication to the company. 'Our workplace cultures reward face time, people who get in early and stay late, people who eat at their desk.'" We value long hours instead of high productivity.[36]

Competitive Disadvantage

In academia and in business, people have to be imported from places where brain function is not yet as undermined by screen culture. This is why China, for example, is quickly growing stronger than the US on every front where there is competition: economic, industrial, academic, technological, and political—American TV-watching is more than double that of the Chinese.[37]

"Our unexpected findings illustrate the secret ingredients of China's economic success, and a serious threat to America's ability to compete in the global marketplace: discipline."[38] This finding focuses on self-management and relationship-management, which require basic building blocks of mental and emotional development lacking in people who grew up watching TV.[39]

It's Not Sentimental

It is a mistake to dismiss the seriousness of our mental and emotional decline as a sentimental "things were better in the good old days" cliché. This change never happened before, from the beginning of human history until the mid-twentieth century.

It is not a case of "people were stronger and more mature in the old days." It is a case of, no matter what decade we're in, if passive screentime is 20,000 hours, we get 20,000 hours less development; if passive screentime is 10,000 hours, we get 10,000 hours less development. It's not to be confused with the proverbial old person's cliché gripe that "the younger generations don't know anything." It is simply the case that for any generation, if passive screentime is 20,000 hours, they will suffer a corresponding impairment in mental function, mental health, and emotional development. This substantial impairment is now scientifically irrefutable, beginning in the mid-twentieth century, and getting worse year after year through today.

No One Is Immune

Older people are not immune to screen damage. Even though some older people had the advantage of more natural, pre-screen, real-life upbringing, later they let their habits degenerate into passive video dependency.[40]

TV's damage is not generation-specific, and not culture-specific. It is human-specific. Lowered brain function is a clinical fact from passive screentime, regardless of age, generation, or region. Anyone in any generation in any culture will suffer the same impairments, and have since the 1950s.

It Doesn't Matter What's On

Studies into TV in particular show that watching TV itself is the problem. It doesn't matter what we watch. The effortless video experience itself deteriorates brain health, and the drug-like pleasantness of it masks the damage as it's happening. Even educational programming delays the child's development.[41] "Numerous studies have found that the actual act of watching TV is even more dangerous and potentially damaging to the brain of the developing child than what's on TV."[42] Regardless of what's on, TV is bad for us and our children.

In an example from Dr. Marie Winn's *Plug-In Drug* ("Sesame Street Revisited"): "Noting that their negative findings about Sesame Street's value were often met with skepticism or outright disbelief by parents of preschool children, the authors offered a number of explanations for parents' refusal to be persuaded that Sesame Street, though a delightful entertainment for young children, does not provide them with a particularly valuable learning experience." "The authors also pointed out the favorable press that Sesame Street had received since its inception."[43]

Parental denial of negative findings about a show they like is to be expected—perception of reality for both parents and children alike has been shaped by immersion in our screen culture.

If a scientific study tells parents that TV is harmful, but a TV publicity campaign tells them that a TV show is good for their kids, parents will reject studies, and believe the TV publicity instead, because it feels better (suggestibility[44]). They deny the science because they like the show. As we saw in the Illusion of Knowledge section earlier, people increasingly reject science as a rule when it is uncomfortable, or threatens their sense of "being right."[45]

The false "reality" is being formed in our brains by screens, while our brain cells are captivated and passive, so it displaces science and facts with whatever feels right or feels good. In the final blow against good judgment, the lowered brain function of the parents actually promotes gross overestimation of their judgment.[46]

For these reasons, "regardless of the content, television has abetted the creation of an increasingly disempowered people who are not only sedentary and dependent upon professionals to entertain them, but are also complacent and acquiescent to the required advertising necessary to pay for the expensive technologies and equipment."[47]

People are comfortable with the idea that TV is bad only because of bad content. But they remain in denial that the real harm is in the medium itself, and has little to do with the content. Some studies reinforce this misdirection of concern by focusing on content only. "Less attention has been paid to the basic allure of the small screen—the medium, as opposed to the message."[48]

Always Passive

Before video entertainment, everyone's brain was naturally active every moment of every day. Screen culture changed that foundational premise of human activity. Now, as a rule, people who watch a lot of video are more passive even while not watching.[49] "Active" was the normal state of a human brain from the beginning of human history until the mid-twentieth century. Today "Passive" is the normal state of the human brain.

Developmental Death Sentence

Being raised in the US today is almost a developmental death sentence. There is indication that universities may be dredging the bottom of the GRE scorers in order to find American-born graduate students, and yet still must take mostly the foreign-born high-scorers in the sciences.[50]

A "new report provides breakdown on international enrollments by discipline and institution, showing that there are graduate STEM programs in which more than 90 percent of students are from outside the U.S."[51]

As facts, evidence, and studies pile higher and higher, showing us how we are destroying ourselves; and as we deteriorate to lower and lower brain function; we also sink deeper into acceptance of our weakened condition and our self-destructive pattern.

Screenlife makes the deterioration process a comfortable one. But it comes at a cost. It is "reported overwhelmingly that today's students have shorter attention spans, are less able to reason analytically, to express ideas verbally, and to attend to complex problems."[52] TV, video, tablet, smartphone and related devices and services are killing us, draining the talent out of our population.

In another study, "The research, which included both elementary school-age and college-age participants, found that children who exceeded two hours per day [of TV] ... were 1.5 to 2 times more likely to be above average in attention problems ... Brain science demonstrates that the brain becomes what the brain does...ADHD is a medical condition, but it's a brain condition ... environmental stimuli can increase the risk for a medical condition like ADHD in the same way that environmental stimuli, like cigarettes, can increase the risk for cancer."[53] TV is exactly the environmental stimulus that increases the risk of harmful brain conditions.

In other research, "the study found that for every extra hour of TV a week the two-year-olds watched there was a 6 percent decrease in math achievement … a 7 percent decrease in classroom engagement, and a 10 percent increase in 'victimization' by peers, such as teasing, rejection and assault. Each extra hour also corresponded with 9 percent less exercise, consumption of 10 percent more snacks, and a 5 percent rise in body mass index … British psychologist Dr Aric Sigman, who has reviewed 30 scientific papers on TV and computer-screen viewing, said that governmental 'advice on TV is conspicuous by its absence. Politicians are scared to take on the entertainment industry, because that industry also provides political news.'"[54]

In this video-entertainment age, all of the forces are conspiring to damage children's brains and distract us from the facts. Parents are the only ones in a position to intervene and give children a better chance at life.

Children's Lost Development

Amazon.com founder and CEO Jeff Bezos credits his success to resourcefulness he learned away from screens, living in the actual world. He spent every summer from age four to sixteen on an isolated farm. There he learned self-reliance, how to build things, how to fix things. "Each time you have a setback, you're using resilience and resourcefulness, and inventing your way out of a box." He passed the same values to his children. Bezos and his wife have "let their kids use sharp knives since they were four and soon had them wielding power tools, because if they hurt themselves, they'd learn. Jeff says his wife's perspective is 'I'd much rather have a kid with nine fingers than a resourceless kid.'"[55]

Nonscreen, real-life playtime is well known to be vital to children's healthy development. NPR's Science correspondent Jon Hamilton brought some of this together, including research from the University of Lethbridge in Alberta, Canada and Washington State University: "The experience of play changes the connections of the neurons at the front end of your brain…those changes in the prefrontal cortex during childhood that help wire up the brain's executive control center, which has a critical role in regulating emotions, making plans and solving problems...The brain builds new circuits in the prefrontal cortex to help it navigate complex social interactions [and we learn] how to interact with others in positive ways...Without play experience, those neurons aren't changed...play is what prepares a young brain for life, love and even schoolwork...the skills associated with play ultimately lead to better grades...But to produce this sort of brain development, children need to engage in plenty of so-called free play. No coaches, no umpires, no rule books...Whether it's rough-and-tumble play or two kids deciding to build a sand castle together, the kids themselves have to negotiate, what are we going to do in this game? What are the rules we are going to follow?"[56]

This crucial emotional development, problem-solving ability, healthy relationships, working with others as an adult, performing well in any occupation, is lost in people who grow up with a lot of TV and video. Essential life skills are disappearing.

The statistics on video-related loss of brain development are overwhelming: the most conservative estimates being 25,000 hours of lost development by age 24, the average probably being closer to 40,000 per 22 years,[57] and perhaps as much as 60,000 hours by age 21.[58]

Based on these facts—men and women in their 20s today barely attain 8-year-old-levels of mental and emotional maturity based on pre-screen standards. The average child today does not develop fundamental life skills, responsibility, caring, fortitude, discipline, intelligence, reasoning, and imagination, among other areas.[59] These facts are so difficult to accept, we subconsciously adopt a collective code of silence on this topic. We just don't talk about it.

Entertainment Casualties

The late-twentieth century's most influential contribution to humanity has been the concept of "Being Entertained."

Entertainment used to be, and should be, the result of active, self-driven, creative effort on the part of people to entertain themselves, as opposed to passively "being entertained" in front of a screen. As a recent *Scientific Learning* article notes, "If we allow children to have poor quality language experiences, substituting entertainment devices for real human language experiences, there will be casualties ... If we allow our children to become socially isolated and distracted by a constant barrage of video entertainment options, there will be casualties."[60]

Reversing the damage requires relearning how to entertain ourselves in ways that require initiative and effort, as it was throughout human history up to the mid-twentieth century. We will have to stop systematically hindering this essential development in our children.

Television Addiction Is No Mere Metaphor

On some level, most people are aware of the effects of TV and other screen devices, but we keep watching, and keep letting our kids keep watching.

People deny they suffer undermining consequences, even while feeling guilty about watching too much. That's why the "common viewer remarks such as: 'If a television is on, I just can't keep my eyes off it,' 'I don't want to watch as much as I do, but I can't help it,' and 'I feel hypnotized when I watch television.'"[61] People often don't enjoy watching TV, but watch it anyway. So it keeps on causing decreased life satisfaction, and increased anxiety.[62]

TV and other screen devices coerce people's minds into the "surrender response." This is the primary feature of addiction.

The pleasure of passive video is so addicting that no decline into low self-esteem, incompetence, and frustration is enough to change the passive-viewing behavior. This is partly because of the self-perpetuating nature of the addiction: Video entertainment forces passivity on the viewer. Being more passive makes the viewer more dependent on video-entertainment for stimulation, and more dependent on video to avoid anxiety. Being more dependent increases the tendency to watch more and more. Watching more and more further increases surrender to passivity and dependence.

"Psychologists and psychiatrists formally define substance dependence as a disorder characterized by criteria that include spending a great deal of time using the substance; using it more often than one intends; thinking about reducing use or making repeated unsuccessful efforts to reduce use; giving up important social, family or occupational activities to use it; and reporting withdrawal symptoms when one stops using it. *All these criteria can apply to people who watch a lot of television.*" The study goes on to say, "Viewing begets more viewing" and "Habit-forming drugs work in similar ways."[63]

Besides hurting ourselves with habitual passive video entertainment, we also hurt our children. Being screen-dependent as parents, we "accept" the mental and physical damage to our children, even while at least partly aware of the negative effects. In a way, shoving screens in front of our children helps us "normalize" the behavior so we feel better about ourselves.

Recent *Washington Post* research cited by Dr. Jim Taylor, an internationally recognized authority on the psychology of sport and parenting, reported that professional basketball players suffer device addiction like the rest of us. "The best basketball players in the world are getting beaten by their phones. They check their phones during team meetings, before games, at half time, and after games. *They know they should stop, but they can't.* Now, apply those same social-media habits to your young athletes and ask yourself whether you think it might be time to help them develop a healthier relationship with their technology."[64]

Professional athletes who provide role models are falling into the same deterioration of skill, discipline, and will, from the same device addiction as everyone else.

In one final, very tragic example from Dr. Marie Winn's "A Chilling Episode" (*Plug-in Drug*), many children were suffering "Tired-Child Syndrome"—"chronic fatigue, loss of appetite, headache, and vomiting"—doctors learned the children were "spending three to six hours of watching television daily, and six to ten hours on weekends." The doctors immediately prescribed removal of TV.

"The effects were dramatic for the 12 children whose parents followed the instructions fully: the symptoms vanished within two to three weeks."[65] It goes on to say the kids whose parents reduced TV but did not eliminate it, achieved proportional partial recovery, or recovery over longer period of time.

The tragic part of the story is that many parents ultimately surrendered to TV at the expense of their children's mental health. Even after witnessing the amazing recovery and renewed health of their children, they later let their children go back to watching. Their children's symptoms returned. The parents put their children on chlorpromazine (antipsychotic medication) to treat the symptoms rather than take the effort to limit TV.[66] Surrender to video addiction was so complete, the parents condemned their own children to a drugged state of helpless brain deterioration, with full knowledge of the inevitable damage to their children.

Weaponized for Addiction

The addiction hooks of electronic devices are designed into the devices and apps to keep users addicted. Adam Alter, author of *Irresistible: The Rise of Addictive Technology and the Business of Keeping Us Hooked*, notes that there are endless user "hooks" embedded in social media, online shopping, and other addictive interfaces. "The list is long—far longer than it's ever been in human history, and we're only just learning the power of these hooks....Compared to the clunky tech of the 1990s and early 2000s, modern tech is efficient and addictive."[67]

The brightest minds in technology today are not helping people deal with technology better—quite the opposite—they are doing everything they can to make the screen takeover our lives, to pull us into irresistible addiction: "According to Tristan Harris, a 'design ethicist,' the problem isn't that people lack willpower; it's that 'there are a thousand people on the other side of the screen whose job it is to break down the self-regulation you have.'"[68]

The intended addictiveness is so effective, experts refer to it as being "weaponized" for addiction: "The people who create and refine tech, games, and interactive experiences are very good at what they do. They run thousands of tests with millions of users to learn which tweaks work and which ones don't—which background colors, fonts, and audio tones maximize engagement and minimize frustration. As an experience evolves, it becomes an irresistible, *weaponized* version of the experience it once was."[69]

Addictive behaviors have become so common they are now mainstream. "These new addictions don't involve the ingestion of a substance ... but they produce the same effects because they're compelling and well designed ... they've all become progressively more difficult to resist."[70] Almost everyone we meet is losing a large part of their life to a screen-related addiction.

Because of a today's almost complete screen immersion, people today experience more brain screenformation, or brain reshaping, than even the previous fifty years of TV and video brain reshaping: "Social media has *completely shaped the brains* of the younger people I work with ... the result is a landscape filled with disconnection and addiction."[71] Our deterioration and addiction is so pervasive, we simply stopped noticing it.

What Technology Leaders Say

In technology circles, the extreme addictiveness of electronic devices, apps, and programs is well known. That's why technology leaders are the ones who most restrict screentime of their own children. They know that the addictiveness is irresistible, and that the addiction will ruin their children's real-life development. Here are some examples:

- "[Steve Jobs] kept the iPad from his kids because, for all the advantages that made them unlikely substance addicts, he knew they were susceptible to the iPad's charms.
- "Evan Williams, a founder of Blogger, Twitter, and Medium, bought hundreds of books for his two young sons, but refused to give them an iPad.

- "Lesley Gold, the founder of an analytics company, imposed a strict no-screen-time-during-the-week rule on her kids.
- "Chris Anderson, the former editor of WIRED, enforced strict time limits on every device in his home, 'because we have seen the dangers of technology firsthand.' His five children were never allowed to use screens in their bedrooms."

"These entrepreneurs recognize that the tools they promote— engineered to be irresistible—will ensnare users indiscriminately."[72]

Smartphones, Social Media, Depression, and Loneliness

Even TV didn't replace in-person relations. It reduced them, but didn't replace them. People couldn't take a TV with them everywhere. Smartphones and tablets let us take TV, games, and social media everywhere we go, and it is deepening the damage to our mental health.

A recent study in clinical psychology found that "adolescents who spent more time on new media (including social media and electronic devices such as smartphones) were more likely to report mental health issues, and adolescents who spent more time on nonscreen activities (in-person social interaction, sports/exercise, homework, print media, and attending religious services) were less likely."[73]

Social media is great for reaching faraway people and staying in touch. But it is a terrible substitute for in-person relationships. "In-person social interaction (also known as face-to-face communication) provides more emotional closeness than electronic communication and … is more protective against loneliness,"[74] whereas, electronic communication, particularly social media, increase feelings of loneliness.[75]

Time spent with electronic devices directly links to suicidal thoughts and clinical depression with in general. As screentime increases, the decline in mental health, the rise in depression, grows steadily worse.

"Since 2010, adolescents spent more time on social media and electronic devices, activities positively correlated with depressive symptoms and suicide-related outcomes. Over the same years, adolescents spent less time on nonscreen activities such as in-person social interaction, print media, sports/exercise, and attending religious services, activities negatively correlated with depressive symptoms [and] iGen adolescents in the 2010s spent more time on electronic communication and less time on in-person interaction than their Millennial and Generation X (GenX) predecessors at the same age."[76] So it is no surprise that iGen in particular are less able to manage stress, fear, and trepidation. These cause exaggerated hesitancy, which keeps them from performing as well as they could.[77]

One way social media depresses us is by tricking us into comparing our real inner self to other people's fake public face. People know they themselves put their best face forward on FB, but forget that everyone else is doing the same thing. The result is depression. Face to Face interaction protects us from this lopsided comparison.

> "If you're feeling bummed, researchers did test for and find a solution. The prescription for Facebook despair is less Facebook. Researchers found that face-to-face or phone interaction — those outmoded, analog ways of communication — had the opposite effect. Direct interactions with other human beings led people to feel better."[78]

Social Media and the Isolation Trap

Unfortunately social media becomes an easy trap for people who are already leading a video-passive lifestyle. It takes some effort to socialize in person. Social media provides an easy alternative to getting up and going out to be with real people. It provides "passive socializing" that fits perfectly with habitually passive lifestyles engendered by our screen culture.

Smartphones and social media complete our isolation from nature, and from each other. TV is proven to be extremely addictive and isolating. But even TV is not nearly as addicting and isolating as today's universal screen-saturation and omnipresent devices. Our

24/7 virtual passivity suffocates us under a state of perpetually downgraded brain function.[79]

As a result of smartphones and social media, people are *never* with people, even when they're nominally "with people." The phenomenon is powerfully depicted in Eric Pickersgill's photo series of people missing out on life, missing out on the joys of being with other people, losing the essence of life-experience that once made us human.[80]

Social media studies are finding similar results: "Facebook use predicts declines in subjective well-being in young adults."[81] As a remedy for screen-related loneliness, we turn to another screen for solace—the social media screen—which merely makes us more lonely and depressed.

Talking to Strangers

The desperation of clinical depression, or just plain loneliness, is a tragic reality that's more prevalent today than ever before.[82] More in-person interaction could improve our mental health, promote a sense of closeness to each other, and reduce loneliness.[83] In the past, this closeness was not just with family and friends, it included talking to strangers.

Before screens isolated us, people felt much more comfortable talking to strangers in public places. It was normal, natural, expected behavior throughout history. Comfortable conversation with strangers gradually became less natural as we became more personally isolated during the mid-to-late-twentieth century. That loss has worsened in recent decades, which undermines our health as a society.

Isolation-related depression didn't happen as much in the past because people got out and visited each other. "In the past, you may go out and meet with your friends and talk about something, but when you got home you'd go to sleep."[84] Today, people might go out to a coffee shop but keep their heads down staring at their smartphone, then go home and spend the evening on social media. Human interaction has no part in it.

A conversation may not cure depression, but the recent spike in loneliness and depression is a direct result of the decline in human interaction. That decline is a direct result of our screen-centric lifestyles, replacing real people with TV, video, and the devices that isolate us.

Physical Contact

Whether talking to strangers, or gathering with friends, physical contact is another part of that interaction which we have lost.

As *Emotional Intelligence 2.0* author and clinical psychologist Travis Bradberry notes, "When you touch someone during a conversation, you release oxytocin in their brain, a neurotransmitter that makes their brain associate you with trust and a slew of other positive feelings. A simple touch on the shoulder, a hug, or a friendly handshake is all it takes to release oxytocin. … Just remember, relationships are built not just from words, but also from general feelings about each other. Touching someone appropriately is a great way to show you care."[85]

A *Clinical Psychological Science* study echoes similar findings: "It is worth remembering that humans' neural architecture evolved under conditions of close, mostly continuous face-to-face contact with others … including touch … and that a decrease in or removal of a system's key inputs may risk destabilization of the system."[86]

As a result of the isolation associated with today's social media, smartphone, TV and general screen culture, people are afraid to touch each other in the healthy human ways that people did for thousands of years until the mid-twentieth century. People are more awkward in any setting of face-to-face interaction. Almost nothing about human interaction comes naturally anymore. Everyone is self-conscious and afraid that everything about human contact is inappropriate because everything about human interaction has become unfamiliar and awkward.

Isolation from people, fewer conversations, and loss of physical contact come with severe deficiencies in emotional development.

These deficiencies produce a host of injuries to our mental health, and "destabilization of the system."

Feeling comfortable striking up a conversation with a stranger, the automatic sense of natural camaraderie with others, and constant daily, even hourly, friendly physical contact, reinforced the feeling that we're all in this together, as well as enhanced brain health. That explains today's decline in people feeling like we're all in this together, as well as the dangerous and pervasive deterioration of mental health.[87]

Company Loves Misery

Comparison on social media engenders a desire to see misfortune in others. People today feel better seeing other people's problems, and feel worse seeing other people's happiness.[88] Is this new prevailing attitude surprising? Consider the factors:

- Video "reality" reduces real-time with friends and reduces exposure to friends' problems.
- Video since childhood leaves us more susceptible to accept video messages as true.[89]
- Social media emphasizes how much more interesting and exciting other people are.
- Isolation prevents corrective, balanced, realistic comparison.
- Social media time correlates to depression and suicidal thoughts.[90]

So when someone posts how they failed at something, people soak it in like nourishment. Finally, someone else has a problem!

The Anxiety Effect

Frequent TV-and-video viewers have worse anxiety as a normal part of their life when away from the screen. Non-viewers or light viewers are happier, and do not experience that anxiety when a screen is not available. Regular viewers require external stimulation at all times. As Robert Kubey notes in his *Scientific American* article, "We wondered whether heavy viewers might experience life differently than light viewers do. ... What we found nearly leaped off the page at us. Heavy viewers report feeling significantly more anxious and less happy than light viewers do in unstructured situations...."[91]

When video-viewers separate from the externally forced "screen structure," and then go into the real world, frustrations become more prevalent, because they no longer possess the ability to cope with life without screen-fed relaxation. They can no longer generate their own brain activity internally. Many people's response to this frustration is to restore temporary brain-comfort with more passive screentime. It becomes a conditioned response to escape the overwhelming anxieties and irritations that arise from normal activity. While it provides an escape, it also further erodes our ability to cope with problems. Life becomes effortless under the calm induced by video-screen stimulation, temporarily. During this passive relaxation, our brain atrophies further.[92]

The Stress Effect

People who watch a lot of TV feel more stress.[93] Having to talk to someone is more stressful, being alone is more stressful. There is no cause for the extra stress, other than a reduced capacity to manage stress. During passive screentime, we are not developing stress-management areas of the brain, like we do when we are more actively engaged in life.

Even when there is nothing stressful in a person's life, TV causes an increase in stress levels. Similar to the anxiety conditioned response, people seek comforting screen entertainment to alleviate stress, not realizing it is a cause. Once again, the act of watching TV increases the need to watch more.[94]

Stress is often associated with having a busy schedule. Screen-related stress creates the illusion of being busy. People claim to be too busy, that life is too hectic, when in fact they are not too busy.

"Most of us are a lot less busy than we claim we are…in general we have 30–40 hours of free time each week…It's very popular, the feeling that there are too many things going on...But the evidence does not back it up."[95]

By spending 30–40 hours a week immersed in passive screentime, the stress becomes real. By wasting all that time, suddenly being busy becomes real.

"No one likes to think of themselves as self-deluded, but the 'busy' trap is easy to fall into…The truth is that we are all much less busy than we think we are. And our consistent insistence that we are busy has created a host of personal and social ills."[96]

The triple-stress from passive video is that it 1. artificially manufactures stress when there is nothing really stressful happening, 2. reduces people's ability to handle stress, and 3. steals so much time that we put things off, miss deadlines, and lose opportunities.

Complaining

We know how annoying it is to hear other people complain. But some of us who complain are not aware of how we are hurting ourselves. It undermines our health, both mentally and physically. Studies show that "complaining makes your synapses make you feel more negative and makes you keep complaining more…" it is also "weakening your immune system; you're raising your blood pressure, increasing your risk of heart disease, obesity and diabetes, and a plethora of other negative ailments."[97]

According to more studies, in addition to sabotaging long-term happiness, the habit of complaining reduces our lifespan by ten or fifteen years.[98]

While we're still alive, complaining keeps us from fixing the very problems we complain about. It is also an ugly habit, pushes other people away, and damages relationships.

Complaints surface more easily when there is less emotional development. Emotional intelligence includes the tools for successful management and healthy processing of irritations, frustrations, and disappointments. This kind of intelligence comes only from an active-minded lifestyle; for example, when the average 21-year-old's screentime of 30,000 or 40,000 hours are replaced with real-life action.

Emotional immaturity causes poor interpersonal relations, such as venting at other people's expense. Subjecting other people to rants demonstrates a self-involved disrespect for other people, and disregard for the relationship. "Emotionally intelligent people place high value on their relationships, which means they treat everyone with respect, regardless of the kind of mood they're in."[99] Emotional intelligence grows only during time spent with people, instead of with screens.

By not complaining, we can actually express our problems more effectively. A complaint is a thoughtless reflex. It makes us feel worse. An expression of problems is a thoughtful conversation. It makes us feel better.

Active minds and emotional intelligence by definition equate to a healthier personality—one that knows how to share the good and bad in life without complaining. Screentime interferes with this kind of healthy brain development. Complaining is simply a less-developed way to process the world.

American author Maya Angelou once said, "Watch yourself about complaining" … "What you're supposed to do when you don't like a thing is change it. If you can't change it, change the way you think about it."[100] She also points out that so-called negatives like hard work become blessings as soon as they're taken away from us. To focus on hardships and neglect blessings is to miss life's opportunities. Once we miss an opportunity, we can't get it back.

How to Be Miserable

Here are ways to make sure we will be miserable. The list below is paraphrased from the article "How To Make Yourself Miserable: Discovering the Secrets to Unhappiness."[101]
- Focus on immediate results and short-term goals.
- Look for quick solutions and expect instant results without putting in any effort.
- Multitask most of the time, and never fully engage in the moment.
- Shift responsibility to others.
- Criticize others while justifying yourself.

- Often compare yourself to others.
- Feel envy.
- Practice victimology—taking the role of victim in the blame game.
- Contemplate the things someone else has done to hurt you.
- Exhibit a bad attitude about most things, events, and people.
- Don't exhibit gratitude.
- Label challenging situations as terrible or horrible.
- Spend time complaining about the way things are.
- Believe you are entitled to anything.
- Resent not getting what you think you're entitled to.

As we have seen up to now, this list aligns with the symptoms of a screen-centric lifestyle.[102]

CHAPTER 2: MANIPULATING PERCEPTION

As the mind is shaped from earliest childhood, our perception forms according to our environment. When our mind is immersed in screens from a young age, perception of the world around us is molded by the medium and its messages. Like the classic fish-in-water analogy, we never stop to question where the water came from, or whether there is a world outside of it. "And the deeper our immersion becomes, the less likely it seems we'll poke our heads above the surface and see there must have been life before someone invented TV."[103] We assume there is no other reality beyond our surroundings.

Screen experience creates our perception of reality, determines what we believe, and defines who we are. Naturally we don't want to believe we have been "brainwashed"—perhaps a better way to put it is that "we are formed and conditioned by an artificial reality that replaced natural development."

Growing up this way leaves us unable to see possibilities of a nonscreen environment, such as life before the twentieth century. We are convinced that our perception of reality, whatever it may be, is the correct perception of reality. Even though the screen weakens our judgment, we will still believe our perception is normal. We have nothing else to compare against.

This long-term screen-based manipulation of perception is not "mind control" like in creepy movies from the 1950s. Screen-centered media does not have to control our minds in any specific way. Instead, the method of screen messaging reshapes our overall perception, judgment, and decision making, over decades of exposure. Growing up with screen-saturated conditioning, our brains function less effectively than would have been the case without the screen-saturated upbringing.

Reshaping Reality into a Consumer Culture

"Consumer Culture" never existed before the 1950s. It was invented by the media. Through the 1950s and 1960s it gradually formed how we think, feel, and view ourselves. It reshaped our perception of what is necessary versus what is optional. "TV has also helped create an increasingly consumerist and considerably helpless people who are thoroughly convinced they must continue buying more and more unnecessary things."[104]

Former luxuries became perceived as necessities by most everyone over the first twenty years of TV. Media invented Consumer Culture and it reshaped us into the Consumers that we have become today. Impulse decision-making for immediate gratification was abnormal until screen culture made it normal.

"Since the mass production of consumer goods requires mass consumption to keep the machines running, television—and thus mass advertising and mass media—has played a leading role in promoting and upholding these values. CEO Lowry Mays of Clear Channel, a media conglomerate with 900 radio stations in the US, plainly stated that 'We're not in the business of providing news and information…We're simply in the business of selling our customers products.' Since television exists in a similar vein of selling what are mostly optional products, it's fair to say then that what television props up is essentially a false economy, arriving under false pretenses."[105]

Most people watch TV and video from age 2 or younger. First and foremost, all media is a tool to create demand—to create a consumer mindset that supports media and increases revenue. All Americans who grew up with TV were shaped by consumption-driven messages that replaced real-life experience. We are formed into passive consumer personalities from infant to adult. "The greatest accomplishment of television then has been to pass itself off as a conveyor of entertainment, news, and occasionally ideas, since its real purpose has been to maintain an audience receptive to commercial advertising … Or rather, *TV doesn't so much advertise products as much as it promotes consumption as a way of life.*"[106]

Once the whole population's perception of reality is reshaped into a consumer mindset, trends in people's decisions and behaviors will fall into place in a predictable way, statistically speaking. Corporations spend $billions on advertisements and on programming, knowing *with certainty* that a predictable percentage will respond as desired.

"By bombarding audiences with an array of subtle and not-so-subtle messages aimed at breeding dissatisfaction in themselves, their cultures and their values, the ultimate goal of television has been to convince people that human needs such as creativity, compassion, understanding, freedom, leisure and security can be replaced and satisfied through material consumption. TV has also helped convince viewers that, when their consumption doesn't seem to be delivering the promised benefits, people just need to consume more."[107]

Our "normal" is the media's creation. Our normal is screen-formed. Our ways of thinking and feeling are conditioned by screen-experience.

Green by Association

With today's proliferation of smartphones, satellites, computers, video games, bigger TVs, more TVs, phones, and automobiles per household than ever, and increases in countless other material goods—we have witnessed a large increase in energy consumption and carbon footprint per person, far beyond the levels that existed in the past (before "going green" was a thing).

Today's intrinsic anti-environmental society didn't just happen. We made it happen because our craving for convenience and entertainment overrode our environmental concerns. Our appetite for consumption was built into our personalities by our lifelong immersion in the screens that form our minds. The formula is simple:

- Screentime makes our minds suggestible.
- Screen media makes us wasteful indulgent consumers.
- Screen media convinces us that we are conscientious environmentalists.

That is our tragic irony. We are the worst environmentalist offenders in history (instilling indulgent consumerist behaviors in us), while feeling a glow of pride over how green we are (reshaping our perception of reality and of ourselves in a way that makes us feel good).

Let's step back for a moment, and take a look at how we got here.

One of the areas where government regulations have benefited society is in stopping the massive dumping of toxic waste, flammable waste, radioactive waste, chemicals like DDT, and other deadly pollution flowing untreated into our aquifers, rivers, lakes, and oceans.

North America was a free, unregulated dumping ground throughout the late 1800s and the early 1900s.

People, on the other hand, wasted almost nothing. There was no plastic, no screens, TV or otherwise. We reused jars, tin cans, fabric, wood. There was no packaging for anything as we know it today. If you want to watch a video, watch this one from National Geographic on how the convenience of plastic has left us drowning in it today.[108] Describing all the differences between today and our pre-plastic past, and all the ways we wasted less in the past, would be a topic for another book. But you get the idea.

Fast-forward to the late twentieth century—a reversal began to happen. Businesses started cleaning up their act, just as regular people began wasting and polluting more.

In the business world, corporate responsibility and energy sustainability have become expected costs of doing business, at least more so than in the past. Companies began promoting themselves using sustainability efforts, promoting reduction of their carbon footprint, and other socially responsible policies.

As we became more "green" in corporate practices, we became more polluted, wasteful, and self-indulgent in our personal lives. The reason is that a passive screen-centric lifestyle makes people self-indulgent and disassociated from the natural world, in ways never before possible. We'll explore several ways this happened later in this section.

Let's start with the most obvious change in the lives of regular people during this period: TV.

"Even if the message on TV is pro-environmental, TV viewing is intrinsically anti-environmental because it provides a substitute for experiencing nature first hand and because it encourages passivity…. In addition, because electronic media are able to make consumer products seem 'more alive than people,' it is inherently biased toward materialistic consumerism…."[109]

In the last thirty years, we started talking more than ever about environmental values, because the screen-messaging told us to. At the same time, we became more wasteful and worse polluters, because screen-messaging said we could. We do what the screen says we can do, and we believe what the screen tells us to believe, even when the two are contradictory.

Screen-messaging told us we are not hypocrites, that we are still environmentally conscientious even while vastly increasing our personal carbon footprints and vastly increasing our damage to the natural world. Screens told us to be more self-indulgent and feel proudly green at the same time. As the screen also destroyed our critical thinking, it was easy for us to embrace this remarkable contradictory fantasy.

We switched from glass to plastic containers, to an endless supply of plastic bags in stores (plastic is an oil product and doesn't decompose easily), started driving more than ever before, owning more cars than ever, profoundly increased our consumer appetite for more luxuries than ever before, including large-carbon-footprint devices such as smartphones. Our habits today make every individual's carbon footprint larger than people thirty years ago could have dreamed possible.[110]

Families today have more cars than families ever had in the past, counteracting the gains from more-efficient engines. In addition to having more cars, we also drive more. We lean on engine technology to justify automobile indulgence, hoping to just about break even. "The single largest source of emissions for the typical household is from driving (gasoline use)."[111]

Today, kids drive or get driven everywhere they go, instead of meeting up with friends and riding bicycles together. For example, kids drive to school, or get driven by their parents. Observe an elementary, middle, or high school in the morning and watch the legions of SUVs dropping off kids. There used to be a legion of bicycles with no parents in sight. Even the wealthiest children in the past would never have dreamed of today's commonplace luxuries. Bicycle-riding kids playing outside with no video devices were much healthier, and represented a truer model of "going green," long before media invented the phrase and fooled us with lies about our greenness.

Today our carbon pollution is double that of 1960.[112]

We use more fossil fuels than ever before. Consumerist messaging from media into screen-saturated personalities made us value material consumption above all other values. That's just the beginning of today's screen-formed fraudulent claims about the value of environmentalism.

Today we take Internet communications and smartphones for granted, which require building, launching, and maintaining satellites to support 24/7 entertainment for everyone. Satellites have become a necessity: "Without them, we wouldn't be able to browse the internet on our phones, send picture messages or make long distance phone calls." They also require earth-based stations to communicate with, and thousands of signal antennas extend signals, and to triangulate to provide GPS information.[113]

Manufacturing, deploying, maintaining, and upgrading of this massive land-air-and-space infrastructure gives us a global carbon footprint beyond the imagination of the 1960s environmentalist teenage protesters. Those same idealistic teenagers of yesterday became just another generation that helped accelerate screen-based consumerism and deceptive messages about "going green" to appease consciences and increase profits. We are all unwitting accomplices.

Today we are green only when convenient, not because we care about *being* conscientious, but because we care about *feeling* conscientious. We pose as environmentally conscientious people because it feels good.

From Meaningful Philosophy to Wealth and Glamour

Another symptom of a video-saturated society is the deterioration of the concept of personal fulfillment. For example, media has changed us from having deeper life values, which would provide authentic fulfillment, to valuing wealth for the sake of being rich, which leaves us empty. Recent research revealed that the "percentage who say it is 'essential' or 'very important' to be 'very well off financially' grew from 41.9% in 1967 to 74.5% in 2005; 'developing a meaningful philosophy of life' dropped in importance from 85.8% in 1967 to 45% in 2005." Additionally, 81% of 18- to 25-year-olds surveyed in a Pew Research Center poll said getting rich is their generation's most important or second-most-important life goal." The *young people themselves* cited the influence of TV shows promoting wealth and glamour as the factors in their outlook.[114]

The fact that passive screentime systematically lowers brain function is clearly proven in every imaginable area of brain activity.[115] Time away from distractions, spent in thoughtful development of values, is yet another casualty. Whether the issue is wealth and glamour, environmental hypocrisy, or embedding consumerist values in general, the cause is our screen-centric lifestyle.

CHAPTER 3: CULTURAL CORRUPTION

A population of active-minded people is prerequisite number one for a healthy society and a vibrant culture. Each mind of each person in a society is a building block of the culture. Our lower-functioning minds from screen-passivity eats away at the fiber of society and the quality of our culture.

We can't fix our culture. It will fix itself if we fix ourselves. But there is a problem: the longer we lead a screen-centric life, the harder it becomes to fix ourselves and to reclaim an active mind.[116] Our minds become increasingly dormant and dependent on screentime. "Thus, the irony of TV: people watch a great deal longer than they plan to, even though prolonged viewing is less rewarding."[117] As a result, developmental building-blocks are lost.

As we lose the basic building blocks of our mental and emotional development, we lose the basic building blocks of our cultural development. To put this in perspective, here are some of the building blocks of our minds and personalities that are lost or damaged by passive screentime[118]:

- Verbal skills
- Math skills
- Intelligence (IQ)
- Emotional intelligence (EQ)
- Maturity
- Imagination
- Attention span
- Concentration
- Critical processing
- Analytical thinking
- Bonding
- Social skills
- Motor skills
- Mechanical skills
- Physical condition
- Overall fulfillment

- Anger and conflict management
- Stability
- Responsibility
- Reliability
- Initiative
- School and work performance
- Ability to hold a job
- Future planning
- Delayed gratification

The greater number of hours spent watching TV, the greater the deficiency in all of these areas.[119]

Cultural corruption follows naturally from deterioration in these areas throughout the population. The only way to address this issue is to convince the population to drastically reduce screentime. This is because there is an inverse relationship between passive screentime and development: as screentime goes up, development goes down. We cannot escape this inverse relationship.

Recipe for Today

It's no surprise that drug abuse and crime increased suddenly and dramatically in the mid-twentieth century. 300,000,000 people dependent on self-destructive behavior is a recipe for evermore destructive tendencies like drug abuse and crime.

TV started in 9 percent of homes in 1950, and increased to 87 percent of homes by 1960.[120] Experts hypothesize all kinds of explanations for drug abuse and crime, but they only address symptoms. The spread of TV alone makes criminal behavior more likely, according to the study reported in "Children who watch 'excessive' amounts of TV are more likely to have criminal convictions, exhibit aggression and experience negative emotions: study."[121]

Aggression comes from a passive mind, not an active mind. A population watching TV doesn't mean everyone becomes a criminal. But it means more people will become criminals. "With every hour in front of the television, kids were more likely to show aggressive behavior or receive a criminal conviction by early adulthood."[122] The rest will just become lower-caliber people.

Decades-long viewing habits have displaced the time that should have been spent developing emotional and mental health. Statistically, a screen-centric society produces more criminals and more crime than a population of non-screen people.

Caring for Others Is Not a Moral Code

As we become more isolated from each other, we become more self centered. Less concern for others is a direct result of less contact with others. Less contact means less familiarity with people, less sharing of life with people, less intimacy with people, less camaraderie. A recent study reported in *Scientific American* showed that in-person interaction is required in order to care about people.[123]

Caring for others is a deep internal process that grows slowly over years spending thousands of hours of personal contact with many people. The interaction-caring correlation is biologically and psychologically linked.

Lack of caring for people is not a mysterious loss of values. It is a law of nature. A rational moral principle that "people should care about each other" is empty and meaningless without time spent with others. The moral code is an after-the-fact idea that follows from how people actually feel. We feel it only by being around people a lot.

So it is an inevitable change in human nature: as contact with others decreases, so caring for others decreases. As isolation increases, so self-centered thoughts, feelings, and behaviors increase.[124] Time with people also determines our focus. More time with others makes us focus on others. More time alone makes us focus on ourselves.

Focus on others makes us better listeners in conversations. We want to ask questions, we show interest. It is not a formula, it is a natural instinct and a true feeling. Time increases interest. We want to get to know each other better, to share in others' experiences.

As *Emotional Intelligence 2.0* author and clinical psychologist Travis Bradberry notes, "To be deliberately empathic, you have to let your ability to walk in their shoes change what you do, whether that's changing your behavior to accommodate their feelings or providing tangible help in a tough situation."[125]

Genuine caring on the inside (as opposed to an "act") goes hand in hand with sharing experiences with one another. It means understanding and caring for people who we disagree with on life choices, religion, politics, social issues, musical taste, and most any issue.

Again, Dr. Bradberry puts it succinctly: "To eliminate preconceived notions and judgment, you need to see the world through other people's eyes. This doesn't require you to believe what they believe or condone their behavior; it simply means you quit passing judgment long enough to truly understand what makes them tick."[126]

This true sense of caring and understanding does not develop in people who lead a screen-centric life. It *cannot* grow where screentime has replaced people time. A screen-dominated personality lacks empathy, which means we cannot understand "caring" as it was once felt.[127]

Caring for others is the *nature of being* for people who grew up spending a lot of time with others. Caring has become another screen-culture casualty.[128]

Homes Filled with Irritable TV Viewers

In families, members grow more distant from one another when they spend time on their separate devices or watch TV—even when they watch TV "together." Home becomes a colder place. Family members are not in touch with other people in the room. They are not interacting.

Viewers are easily irritated when someone in the room starts talking. This is because of the Alpha/Beta Wave switch that we learned about in the first chapter of this book. The brain shifts to sleeplike Alpha Waves while watching TV, and is jarred back into

Beta Waves to engage with the person talking.[129] The shift irritates us when we are in the sleep-like Alpha state, like an unwelcome alarm clock going off. Instead of greeting a loved one entering the room, we snap at them for disrupting our hypnotic TV-viewer state of passivity.

TV Makes Us Miserable and then Kills Us

In addition to undermining our mental and emotional development, TV undermines physical health. "There's no shortage of research showing links between watching too much television and early death.

- "Every hour of television you watch reduces your life expectancy by close to 22 minutes.
- "The researchers found people who watched more than three hours of television a day had double the risk of premature death when compared to those who watched less than one hour per day.
- "But when they looked at other sedentary behaviors—driving a car and using a computer—they didn't find the same links with early death."[130]

What's special about the findings is that other sedentary behaviors don't have the same death-correlation as watching TV. *TV specifically damages health, over and above the negative impact of sedentary behavior in general.*

It gets worse. Every year TV-viewing is linked to 1,140,480 new cases of diabetes, 246,240 additional deaths from heart disease, and 673,920 additional deaths. "Evidence from a spate of recent studies suggests that the more TV you watch, the more likely you are to develop a host of health problems and to die at an earlier age."[131]

- "In a new analysis published … in the Journal of the American Medical Association, researchers combined data from eight such studies and found that for every additional two hours people spend glued to the tube on a typical day, their risk of developing type 2 diabetes increases by 20% and their risk of heart disease increases by 15%.

- "The increased risk of disease tied to TV watching 'is similar to what you see with high cholesterol or blood pressure or smoking'
- "The findings are remarkably consistent across different studies and different populations
- The studies "included more than 175,000 people around the world and generally lasted between 6 and 10 years....most controlled for a long list of health factors (such as body mass index, cholesterol levels, and family history of disease) in an effort to pinpoint the effect of TV watching."[132]

Again, these studies *rule out sedentariness alone*, and other factors, and *specifically pinpoint TV as the direct cause of death and disease*.

We Are the Rats

Studies cited in this book have provided the science and the proof that the population has been damaged, weakened, corrupted, and in many cases killed, by screentime—and that we are largely unaware of this correlation or this damage. The disease of passivity and arrested development has spread across hundreds of millions of people over several generations. It has resulted in a less-capable, less-mature, less-stable, less-healthy population.

Our society has become an experiment of video-immersion on mental and physical health. Short term screen-fed rewards feel good, which prevents us from noticing the side-effects of mental and physical damage (similar to heroin in a rat). We are left wanting more.

In the experiment, the screens that give the temporary "high" are controlled to prevent us from learning the long-term damage. Then we are fed the self-deception that we are still in control of our own values and decisions, while repeated reinforcements guide our behavior.

We have become like the lab rats following the guided behavior. We became incapable of critical self-knowledge, because those functions were systematically disabled by the screen-drug. The result is pervasive mental and physical deterioration in a population of easily conditioned rats in a maze of screens.

Words of Warning

Words of warning don't get to the public because we rely on the culprit itself for our information. If what we learn comes from screens, we will not learn about screen-related damage. TV-and-video information merely creates an illusion of being informative, while it feeds "guided reality" into minds made suggestible by the medium itself.[133]

As noted scholar and *The Death of Expertise* author Tom Nichols points out: "Just as clicking through endless Internet pages makes people think they're learning new things, watching headlines is producing laypeople who believe—erroneously—that they understand the news. Worse, their daily interaction with so much media makes them resistant to learning anything more that takes too long or isn't entertaining enough."[134]

If we continue informing ourselves from screen-sources, we will become less informed, and less aware of the deficiency. Changing our behavior is the only way to change the consequences.

For example, damage from excessive Alpha Wave state passivity can be reversed, but only by eliminating or significantly reducing screentime. This kind of lifestyle change has been rewarding for many people, and worth the struggle. But it can be very difficult at first. For example, in a Kubey and Csikszentmihalyi study "Television Addiction is no mere metaphor": At first, where families try eliminating TV, "family members had difficulties in dealing with the newly available time, anxiety and aggressions were expressed.... People living alone tended to be bored and irritated."[135] These are typical symptoms of addiction withdrawal: anxiety, aggression, irritation. But after the first few weeks, symptoms are reduced and people begin leading healthier lives, mentally and physically. This might be the most important life-changing struggle we ever decide to undertake.

CHAPTER 4: EDUCATIONAL CORRUPTION

Many people believe that Americans value "learning how to think for ourselves" and that the American education system teaches students how to think for themselves. While it is comforting to feel that we attain this ideal of educational value, the facts are less comforting.

We know that Americans watch more TV than most cultures and that TV prevents independent thinking, undermines logical processing, lowers IQ, and makes brains more suggestible to being influenced by external messages.[136]

Based on Nielsen and other studies, the average American spends between 25,000 and 60,000 hours passively watching TV by their early 20s[137]—so their minds less developed by that number of hours. Adults who grew up watching average amounts of TV, including educators, have suffered the same damage to cognitive function, have lower functioning brains, and are underdeveloped overall. These are the standard conditions proven to be widespread in today's population,[138] and the public schools are no exception. They simply reflect universally lower standards and capabilities that reflect today's norms and are today's reality.

Since the 1960s, teachers increasingly have compensated for students' shorter attention spans and weakening concentration by trying to "make learning fun." Teachers are supposed to "get students excited" about learning. This compensation for deficiencies merely nurtures passivity and failure.

By exaggerated nurturing and over-protectiveness, we send the message that mental comfort is more important than mental development. But why can't we have both? We can't have both because mental comfort and mental development are mutually exclusive. Learning requires discomfort, it has to be hard in order to be successful. We want to "stretch our boundaries" and "reach outside our comfort zone," and so we should. We should also push students to learn that lesson.

Instead, we train students to resent hard work. We prevent them from reaching beyond their comfort zone. As *The Death of Expertise* author Professor Tom Nichols warns, "the protective, swaddling environment of the modern university infantilizes students and thus dissolves their ability to conduct a logical and informed argument. When feelings matter more than rationality or facts, education is a doomed enterprise."[139]

Brain development requires strenuous exercise just as muscle development requires strenuous exercise (this is developed more fully in the "Like a Muscle" section of this book). If it is not painful, it is not learning.

Improvement should be its own reward. As *The Motivation Myth* author Jeff Haden aptly points out, "Improving feels good. Improving breeds confidence…so you naturally want to keep improving."[140] One of the best lessons in life is that "my aversion to 'hard' goes away once I break a sweat."[141] When "hard" is not required, the lesson is never learned.

Teachers should explain subjects, assign work, and test progress. Students should listen quietly and attentively, do their homework, study for tests, and perform. Set expectations. Do the painful deed or fail. Then enforce it. Students who fail to do their work are supposed to fail.

We hear this simple formula, roll our eyes, and say "Get real." This simple process sounds farfetched today, even though it was done precisely this way, with consistent success, for hundreds of millions of students, for hundreds of years, until the latter twentieth century, when TV began lowering mental functions and educational expectations. Today, the main truth learned is that learning is not part of the educational program.

Mocking Ourselves because Math Is Hard

Instead of valuing complex learning in all areas of the mind, our culture has sunk into a kind of surrender, celebrating getting dumber and dumber. The decline and the surrender show up in social media tropes, on T-shirts, in ads, saying things like "Poetry is hard,

Mmmm Bacon" or "Math is Hard, Let's go Shopping." Sure, these are funny at first. And people say, "It's just a joke." Yet it accurately reflects today's mindset and skillset. It expresses our cultural values.

Far from being funny, it is sickening to see the population self-administering brain deterioration, surrendering, and laughing.

One way to adapt to a lower functioning "math-is-hard" attitude is to remove math requirements. We adapt by accepting the deterioration, for example, in programs like a San Francisco Middle School approach to simply remove Algebra 1 from the curriculum.[142]

Everyone chuckles and says, "Hey, I'm no good at math," with a wink that says, "Nobody cares anyway." Like the example given in the article "We're evil, and proud of it," TV ads mock the idea of TV melting our brains even though the actual deterioration of the brain is happening while advertisers and viewers laugh at the joke together.[143]

An 'A' for Everyone

Students are being fooled into thinking they are exceptional, by the sharp increase in A's being handed out in schools, K–12, public or private, and in Ivy League and State Colleges.

Easy A's didn't start in the 2000s, or the 1990s. The first sharp increase in handing out A's happened from the late 1960s to the early 1970s—exactly when the first generation of kids who grew up with TV entered the educational system.[144]

This is one of dozens of similar TV-effects that surfaced at that same time, for the same reason. It was the first generation that was "made stupid" by too much TV.[145]

Disproportionate awarding of A's has continued to rise steadily since the 1970s. And as Catherine Rampell's *Washington Post* article points out:

- "A's—once reserved for recognizing excellence and distinction—are today the most commonly awarded grades in America.
- "That's true at both Ivy League institutions and community colleges, at huge flagship publics and tiny liberal arts schools,

and in English, ethnic studies and engineering departments alike. Across the country, wherever and whatever they study, mediocre students are increasingly likely to receive supposedly superlative grades.

- "Analyzing 70 years of transcript records from more than 400 schools, the researchers found that the share of A grades has tripled, from just 15 percent of grades in 1940 to 45 percent in 2013"[146]

It's not because students are "doing better than ever." Students in the US are doing worse than ever. As Ray Williams' *Psychology Today* article notes: "After leading the world for decades in 25-34 year olds with university degrees, the U.S. is now in 12th place."[147] While we fool ourselves with more A's than ever, with absurd GPAs like 4.9 on a 4.0 scale, the rest of the world is leaving us in the dust.

More warning signs of our doing worse than ever come from a recent Educational Testing Service (ETS) report: "Indeed, while millennials are often portrayed in the media as being on track to be our best educated generation ever, their skill levels are comparatively weak." As compared with the same age group in other countries, "the comparatively low skill level of U.S. millennials is likely to test our international competitiveness over the coming decades. If our future rests in part on the skills of this cohort—as these individuals represent the workforce, parents, educators, and our political bedrock—then that future looks bleak."[148]

The warning signs of our descent continue as the *New York Times* reports from the Organization for Economic Cooperation and Development, the US scores 17th in numeracy testing, among 16- to 29-year-olds with a bachelor's degree. "While results vary somewhat depending on the subject and grade level, America never looks very good. The same is true of other international tests. In PISA's math test, the United States battles it out for last place among developed countries, along with Hungary and Lithuania."[149]

Professor Tom Nichols points out the detriment to students: "Colleges and universities also mislead their students about their own competence through grade inflation. Collapsing standards so that schoolwork doesn't interfere with the fun of going to college is one way to ensure a happy student body and relieve the faculty of the pressure of actually failing anyone."[150]

As passing out A's like candy increases, reward becomes more disconnected from performance. Students are trained to feel entitled to an A grade as a matter of course. "Professors marvel at the way students now shamelessly demand to be given good grades, regardless of their work ethic, but that's exactly what you would expect if the student views themselves as a consumer, and the product as a credential, rather than an education."[151]

If students' self-esteem is temporarily propped up by fraudulent GPAs, it will be mercilessly torn down by real-life competition later. That's not doing students a favor, it's a cruel trick being played on them. Some rationalize that exaggerated grades nurture students' self-esteem. Instead, as Rampell notes, we are "hampering the ability of students to compete in the global marketplace."[152]

To be fair, many teachers are under pressure to give exaggerated grades. That trail leads back to money, with funding based on school performance (such as average GPAs or graduation rates), whereas true student development is not part of the equation.

Administrators are under similar pressure to put pressure on teachers, for the same reasons. In some cases their livelihoods and careers are at stake: deliver high grades to get more funding. Students are the losers. When we put our kids' learning into the hands of bureaucrats competing for money, this is what we can expect.

At the college level, there are even more politics at play. Graduates with higher GPAs and more honors are more likely to get job placement, regardless of the lack of real learning. That means colleges can say more of their students get jobs in their field of study, which attracts more new students, which increases revenue. It's a business. As Nichols warns, the commoditization of degrees, and the insatiable demand to keep printing more of them, at the overstressed assembly lines of diploma mills in America, we're descending into a destructive spiral of credential inflation.[153]

Whether K-12, public or private; or college, Ivy League or State School; student performance is the least significant factor in the grades they receive, and the least significant factor in our educational policies.

Educational deterioration and commoditization traces back to greed, negligence, immediate gratification, artificial self-esteem, and lower functioning minds enacting policies that work against intellectual development. This is evident in government, in colleges, in public schools.

Corruption is nothing new. But what is new, is the massive scale of this fraud beginning in the 1960s and 1970s, which never happened before in history, and which continues to get worse today.

Other countries are starting to imitate American poor performance. For example, in Britain: "An international survey by the Organisation for Economic Cooperation and Development has found standards of literacy and numeracy among school-leavers in England and Northern Ireland to be among the lowest in the developed world. Shockingly, older people leaving the workforce were better educated than those joining it. This may be the first time in recorded history that such a phenomenon has occurred, with the young worse educated than their parents."[154] As other countries drop to US levels of screen-related lower functioning, we will witness the spread of educational deterioration.

A College Eye View

From this author's firsthand experience both as a graduate student and as a university administrator, colleges are requiring less and less of their students. As *The Death of Expertise* author Professor Tom Nichols noted, "In the worst cases, degrees affirm neither education nor training, but attendance. At the barest minimum, they certify only the timely payment of tuition," and adds that "students now graduate believing they know a lot more than they actually do," while "Intellectual discipline and maturation have fallen by the wayside."[155]

Colleges and Universities are places to make special memories of youthful carefree years, but not necessarily places of rigorous development of any kind.

Between two students with the same degree from the same college, with the same GPA, there might be one with very little learning, and another with a lot of learning. Requirements for assignments, and standards for "passing a class," are a lot lower than in the past. Required reading has become less challenging. There is a steady and systematic reduction of difficulty. As Nichols observes, "Less is demanded of students now than even a few decades ago. There is less homework, shorter trimester and quarter systems, and technological innovations that make going to college more fun but less rigorous. When college is a business, you can't flunk the customers."[156]

As a result, the lesser-learning student can easily graduate with the same degree as the student who learns a lot. Nichols echoes this new fact of college education today: "'College graduate' today means a lot of things. Unfortunately, 'a person of demonstrated educational achievement' is not always one of them."[157] Graduates not only fail to achieve expertise in anything, they even don't learn enough to *recognize* expertise in others.[158]

For those students who want to learn more, who appreciate the sacrifice and the rewards of painful effort and fulfillment, who know learning has nothing to do with entertainment, who push themselves to learn on their own, the university can provide guidance and resources.

Universities still have dedicated mentors, old-school professors, just waiting for a few students who want something more from college. Those professors will devote extra time to work with those students, to make the diploma stand for something more substantial. But that kind of accomplishment is no longer required in order to receive a diploma. It doesn't make the piece of paper, it just makes the piece of paper meaningful.

There is some good news: Some colleges are changing admissions tests to filter out students with spoiled attitudes, to get a higher proportion of more driven students. Psychological testing showing an attitude of "I've got to put in more effort" instead of "It's the professor's fault I'm not learning" might open more doors to get into college ahead of others with a higher GPA from high school.[159]

Another idea that might improve the college-student population is a 13th Grade option offered at some Oregon high schools. It is an optional "super senior" year, grade 13. It's an option for students who want to learn, and it counts towards college:

"The program gets its money—and its legality—from allowing the 13th-graders to exist in a sort of definition limbo: They've technically completed high school, but they're not given diplomas yet, which grants them continuing eligibility for the state's $6,500-per-student allowance—which, it turns out, is enough money to pay for community college tuition, books and lab fees, and have a substantial chunk of change left over for all that support and oversight. Then once they finish the 13th grade, students get that diploma and they can enter college as sophomores."

Comparing it to the European extra year of preparation and testing to ensure college readiness:

"They also have the intellectual maturity that can only come from the protracted preparation for something that, quite unlike the SAT and our current No Child Left Behind tests, is truly nuanced and demonstrative of true scholarly inquiry and progress—you know, like work in college is supposed to be."[160]

It might just be another program that fails to address the root cause of ill-prepared students whose minds are already too passive by age 18. But as an already-funded option to identify and help serious learners, it's a start. As Schuman notes:

"Wherever you stand on the political spectrum, unless you are truly delusional, you must admit that the American K-12 system is currently ... underperforming, and could use ... a 'creative disruption'."[161]

Guilty Overparenting

When video lifestyles and screen-centric habits separate and isolate parents from children, parents are less attuned to issues in the life of a child. They miss opportunities to help, opportunities that would have fostered natural parent-child bonding.

Screen-related parent-child estrangement has become a common form of neglect, beginning in the mid-twentieth century and worsening every decade since. Parents often try to compensate for the distance that they caused, by lavishing too much sympathy on their children's tiniest troubles.

Over-attention reveals being out of touch just as much as under-attention. Over-attention is an exaggerated attempt to "show they care" for a moment. It is forced and unnatural against the lack of bonding from screen isolation. Over-parenting leaves kids with escalated anxiety when faced with challenges in the real world.[162]

Parents also compensate for lack of quality time together by over-serving kids, especially while they are watching TV. It becomes a habit, and an expectation, and another developmental impediment that undermines the child's ability to grow up.[163]

Additionally, parents damage their children with over-praising minor accomplishments, with disproportional accolades. Their children grow up to expect exaggerated rewards. "While experts say it's natural for humans to seek attention, these young people revel in it. They're accustomed to being noticed, having been showered with awards and accolades."[164]

Overparenting is now continuing into kids' late teens and young adulthood. Today, parents take care of their kids' college applications, financial aid forms, bank accounts, job-search, and give them credit cards. Some parents even want to be present at their adult kids' job interviews (a humiliation that causes further estrangement). Meanwhile, overparenting undermines the young adult's coping skills, and further delays the young adults' ability to competently function in the real world.[165]

Attraction to the Difficult

Throughout history, people thrived on tough, painful mental and physical challenges. Normally developed minds feel a strong attraction to difficult hurdles, pursuing them with determination and enthusiasm.

During the mid- to late-twentieth century, when screen-formed minds replaced naturally formed minds, we began losing interest in the difficult. We reshaped into a preference for whatever is easiest. Passive screen entertainment gave us this way of life, which has weakened us ever since. Instead of energy to meet challenges, we have numbness and remain passive.[166]

The fact alone that the average American watches 30 to 40 hours of TV per week, plus many more hours with other screen-device entertainment, is itself an attraction to the easy and effortless. That fact alone proves our switch from active and strong to passive and weak. No other activity or lack of activity or any other comparison or evidence is necessary to prove the point. This fact *by itself* proves that we lost active time and gained passive time.

If earlier people had TV, they would have deteriorated just as today's people have deteriorated. They would have succumbed to the same passive dependency. Fortunately for them, they were not immersed in a screen culture, so they developed more, and led more active lives.

Unfortunately for us, we are surrounded by video entertainment and smart devices that make us dumber. We are left with lower-functioning brain patterns and a culture of lethargy and apathy. Removing TV and other video entertainment is the only way to fix it.[167]

One of the greatest gifts we could ever give to ourselves and to others, is to switch back to a natural, active lifestyle. Truer words were never spoken, than these by *The Motivation Myth* author Jeff Haden: "All of our success and growth comes from choosing the hardest and least comfortable way."[168]

Like most effort-related discomfort: "After the first few times you lean into your discomfort, you will quickly find that the discomfort isn't so bad, it doesn't ruin you, and it reaps rewards."[169]

Multitasking

As new behaviors grow more common in society, we have to create a label for them. As screentime systematically attacks our ability to concentrate, and kills our attention spans, the behavioral symptoms of this breakdown need a label. The label we gave to one symptom of lost attention span is "multitasking."

Multitasking is a behavior pattern derived from the passive screen-culture of hectic-but-ineffectual movement that passes for activity. The loss of concentration and attention span compromises our effectiveness when dealing with a multitude of tasks. What people call "multitasking" (e.g., having several assignments going at the same time, rapidly switching between tasks) makes people less effective, wastes time, and reduces the quality of everything we do. The mind functions at a lower level when multitasking. "Multitasking actually sacrifices your quality of work, as the brain is simply incapable of performing at a high level in multiple activities at once."[170]

No matter how young and energetic, or no matter how old and experienced, multitasking yields inefficiency, missed deadlines, stress, and poor results. It has become an excuse for cheapness and low quality. Multitasking is a fragmented mode of limited surface engagement, symptomatic of easily distracted brains.[171]

"Ultra-productive people know that multitasking is a real productivity killer. Research conducted at Stanford University confirms that multitasking is less productive than doing a single thing at a time. The researchers found that people who are regularly bombarded with several streams of electronic information cannot pay attention, recall information or switch from one job to another as well as those who complete one task at a time."[172]

Focusing on big chunks of work, and staying with it until it's done, will reduce stress and headaches. It will improve quality and productivity in the short run and in the long run.

Old School Note Taking

Computers can be used for mentally active purposes, whereas watching videos almost never can be a mentally active experience. But even when we think a computer is helping us learn, it might actually be slowing us down.

A study using undergraduates from UCLA and Princeton, showed students taking notes on a laptop score significantly lower than students who took notes by hand. When the test was a half-hour after the note taking, they scored about the same in the fact-based questions, but laptop students score poorly on conceptual questions, while handwritten note takers scored well.

Testing a week later, laptop students scored poorly on both fact-based and conceptual questions, while handwritten note takers scored well in both areas.[173]

Note taking is an important way to develop the mind and learn more effectively. It turns out that how we take notes makes a difference. Even when screens are used actively as a learning tool, non-screen methods enable deeper conceptual learning and better retention than the same activity on a screen device.

Reading Good Books Enhances and Lengthens Life

Great works of fiction are those with a more layered, complex investigation into the human condition, written in an artistic language resulting from painstaking development, so that it appears effortless.

Reading is a demanding process that yields deeper pleasure and more meaningful experience than movies and video. Every good book we read creates more depth in our thinking.

We also gain a deeper understanding of other people: "an influential study published in *Science* found that reading literary fiction (rather than popular fiction or literary nonfiction) improved participants' results on tests that measured social perception and empathy, which are crucial to 'theory of mind': the ability to guess with accuracy what another human being might be thinking or feeling."[174]

It turns out we can enjoy our books longer as well, because reading them makes us live longer, according to another study: "Overall, the researchers calculated that book reading was associated with an extra 23 months of survival. … Reading magazines or newspapers didn't have the same effect ... it's the deep engagement required by the narrative and characters of fiction, and the length of both fiction and nonfiction books, that increases cognitive skills and therefore extends lives."[175] Reading lengthens life (and improves the quality of it); watching TV shortens life[176] (and destroys the quality of life). What a choice.

Homeschooling

Hope for tomorrow comes from involved parents, who supplement school with home education (or just homeschool altogether), who stop letting kids watch TV, and minimize any kind of screen exposure on any device.

For those who still question the efficacy of homeschooling, here are a few facts from a recent study:
"The study included almost 12,000 home-school students from all 50 states who took three well-known standardized achievement tests…The students were drawn from 15 independent testing services, making it the most comprehensive home-school academic study to date.

- "In reading, the average home-schooler scored at the 89th percentile; language, 84th percentile; math, 84th percentile; science, 86th percentile; and social studies, 84th percentile. In the core studies (reading, language and math), the average home-schooler scored at the 88th percentile.
- "The average public school student taking these standardized tests scored at the 50th percentile in each subject area.

- "The average home-school test results continue to be 30-plus percentile points higher than their public school counterparts.
- "In a sentence, home-schooling is a recipe for academic success."[177]

Most people would like to see public education be the best option to prepare kids for the real world. But at present public education is the worst option.

How Our Presidents Represent Us

The steadily decreasing aptitude of the US population is reflected in the declining literacy of presidential speeches. It provides yet another reference point that reflects the mental decline of Americans and correlating it to the TV timeline.

Tracking trends over the course of 600 presidential speeches, starting with George Washington, up to the second term of Barak Obama, the trend shows a steady decline.[178] One attempt to explain it is to say presidents spoke to voters, and in the early 1800s, only well-off landowners could vote. With a broader voting public, the argument says, literacy of speeches had to be lowered to communicate. But that argument doesn't explain it.

Education has never been more broadly available to everyone, K–12, than it is today. How people use their educational opportunity, and the quality of institutions of education, are what make the difference.

In 1800, even landowners were often "uneducated" in the sense that they didn't get much formal schooling. Yet they possessed much higher reading levels and aptitude than today's graduates. Self-taught reading-and-learning lifestyles were common. For example, George Washington had a "meager education"—he "never received more than the equivalent of an elementary school education [and was] not highly literate."[179]

George Washington had a meager elementary school education and was not highly literate by eighteenth and nineteenth century standards, but his speeches were at today's Ph.D. reading level.

Twenty-first century speeches average about 9th grade.

There is a steady record of graduate-level presidential speeches in the eighteenth and nineteenth centuries. The only time someone like Thomas Jefferson spoke below today's college level was speaking to people who knew English only as a second language, such as his 1806 speech to the Cherokee Nation (8th-grade level), or his 1803 speech to the Choctaw Nation (10th-grade level). George Washington spoke to the Cherokee and Seneca Nations closer to 11th-grade level.[180]

People with no school whatsoever, who knew English only as a second language, had equal or higher reading levels than today's mass educated culture.

Speeches to English-speaking American citizens remained at today's college level to Ph.D. level until the twentieth century. In the past, the general public made themselves more literate than people today, with much less formal schooling than today. Adults taught children or they learned on their own.

To achieve such levels of learning without formal education, they must have appreciated delayed gratification, long-term rewards of painful study. No one forced them to go to school and sit through class. They wanted the pain, because they understood the gain. They had the initiative on their own, and they cherished higher functioning as an important value.

The real drop in presidential-speech reading levels begins in the 1920s as radio starts to replace reading as an information source. Public literacy drops more dramatically and rapidly after TV hit the scene. It is reflected in the drop in presidential-speech literacy to 9th-grade levels by the late twentieth century, where they remain today.[181]

Confirmation Bias

Of the many ways screentime has compromised us, confirmation bias and the related tendency of self-segregation are two ways that don't get enough attention.

The increase of screenlife with smartphones and social media has heightened our susceptibility to "close ranks" socially, a voluntary tendency towards self-segregation. Screenlife makes it easy to exclude people and comments that we don't already believe and love. As *The Death of Expertise* author Tom Nichols observes, "the Internet has politically and intellectually mired millions of Americans in their own biases. Social media outlets such as Facebook amplify this echo chamber." Even if we don't intentionally block what we disagree with, Facebook feeds us what we "like" as part of its service.[182] We segregate from differing people as well as from differing information sources. By replacing social life with social media, we reduce or remove exposure to differing views.

Relying on the Internet for research, news, and information reinforces our mistaken ideas and biases. There are no signposts to tell us which sites are truly peer-reviewed scientific sources, or rigorous high-caliber journalism; versus poorly substantiated "sciencey" sites, yellow journalism, or flagrant misinformation. Instead of searching for truth, we search to confirm our pre-existing opinions, auto-select sources we like, and hear what we want to hear.

The name for this behavior is *confirmation bias*. "Once we have formed a view, we embrace information that confirms that view while ignoring, or rejecting, information that casts doubt on it.…We pick out those bits of data that make us feel good because they confirm our prejudices."[183] Confirmation bias is operating when we:

- Overlook bad arguments if they support our beliefs
- Ignore faulty logic if we feel good about the conclusions
- Don't bother to investigate an experiment if we agree with the results
- Accept what we like, and reject what we don't like, regardless of the truth.

By definition, confirmation bias means we can always feel right about everything we think.

The Internet, TV, and other screen-media promote confirmation bias, which further segregates society. "Today, there is a news source for every taste and political view, with the line between journalism and entertainment intentionally obscured to drive ratings and clicks." Furthermore, we choose our sources according to our bias, "people gravitate toward sources whose views they already share."[184] News channels must chase oversimplified political demographics to make money for their advertisers. The media promotes artificial divisions between us, which gradually become real divisions between us. We are molded by what we watch, we segregate ourselves accordingly.

Here we see the vicious cycle of screen-centric news and information:

- Oversimplified biased reporting that promotes hostility and division to woo the "liberal market" or the "conservative market" to make money, instead of neutral objective reporting, which doesn't win ratings or make money.
- Uncritical acceptance (if you already agree) and uncritical rejection (if you already disagree) of the message: confirmation bias.
- Self-perpetuated social segregation.

To use the congressional metaphor, both sides of the aisle are equally guilty of confirmation bias. According to recent studies, conservatives and liberals alike reject evidence if it contradicts their values. Both will discount science when it challenges their worldview.[185]

This trend will continue to worsen as long as we absorb information from screens. Passively watching the news on a screen makes us much more susceptible to confirmation bias. As shown earlier, TV shuts down the brain's logical processing faculties. We are merely absorbing and feeling, instead of processing and thinking. If the infotainment feels good, then it's true; if it feels bad, then it's false. In today's world of screenformation, we yell reactively "I'm right!" In the past world of objective information gathering, we spoke thoughtfully, "I'll try to understand your opposing view."

CHAPTER 5: EXERCISE, ANGER AND FIGHTING

There are endless, seemingly infinite, numbers of studies showing us how important it is to exercise regularly and rigorously. For example, there is only one way to create new brain neurons for a sharper mind later in life: "new neurons are produced in the brain throughout the lifespan, and, so far, only one activity is known to trigger the birth of those new neurons: vigorous aerobic exercise."[186]

Thirty minutes a day of focused painful exercise immediately promotes mental energy and physical energy. It provides deeper peace of mind, a more balanced flow of serotonin and other healthy brain chemicals, a stronger more focused mind, increased clarity and alertness, stronger heart, less chance of heart attack or stroke, increased sexual ability, better circulation, reduced toxins, reduced likelihood of diabetes, reduced likelihood of cancer, stronger immune system, better and deeper sleep every night (again boosting immunity), easier time waking up every morning, and less physical discomfort doing everyday activities—plus a happier, stronger, sharper mind.[187]

As *Emotional Intelligence 2.0* author and clinical psychologist Travis Bradberry notes, "None moreso than vigorous exercise … releases chemicals in your brain like serotonin and endorphins that recharge it and help to keep you happy and alert. They also engage and strengthen areas in your brain that are responsible for good decision-making, planning, organization, and rational thinking."[188]

In addition to specific routines, we can supplement formal exercise with choices such as taking the stairs instead of the escalator or elevator, if at all possible. Taking the stairs improves brain function and neuronal health ("brain age decreases…by 0.58 years for every daily flight of stairs climbed").[189] While taking the stairs is not possible for many people, for those who are fortunate enough to have that choice, it is foolish not to take it.

While we're at it, brain exercises also enhance brain health. One particular point proven in recent years is that mental exercise prevents memory loss, Dementia, Alzheimer's, senility, and mental deterioration in general. Conversely, TV viewing is an indicator of these diseases. Step one: Stop watching TV.[190]

Let us review the consequences of the short-term easy path of lethargic inactivity: escalated anxiety, deeper depression, fewer brain neurons, less energy, a weaker less-focused mind, dementia, unbalanced brain-chemical flow, deficient sexual abilities, weaker heart, greater risk of heart attack and stroke, increased likelihood of cancer and diabetes, reduced circulation, weaker immune system, troubled sleep, a harder time getting out of bed every morning, disorganization, irrational thinking, and more physical discomfort doing everyday activities.

The main obstacle keeping most of us from the active healthy path is screen dependency, or indirectly through screen-induced laziness, which steals our time and drains our energy.

Angry Reaction

A screen-centric lifestyle indirectly breeds impatience and shortens tempers. This is because screentime gradually makes our minds more passive. One definition of passive mindedness is the lack of ability to effectively process irritations and aggravations, both large and small. Thus short-temperedness is predicted by a passive mind.

Another definition of passive mindedness is less exertion of mental effort. It takes effort (active mind) to process experiences effectively. Failure to exert effort, and failure to process experiences effectively, follow from a screen-centric lifestyle. It has become axiomatic that growing up watching too much TV leads to this kind of failure.[191]

A screen-symptom similar to short-temperedness is bitterness. The emotional marriage from hell is the marriage of bitterness and stress—and they are typically found together. It signals an almost complete failure to develop the faculty called Emotional Intelligence, or EQ. Bitter people, who do not process anger very well, suffer greater stress. As clinical psychologist Travis Bradberry notes, "Researchers at Emory University have shown that holding onto stress contributes to high blood pressure and heart disease. Holding onto a grudge means you're holding onto stress, and emotionally intelligent people know to avoid this at all costs."[192]

Bitter, stressed, short-tempered people are pushed around by events (passive) instead of taking command of the moment by processing events (active). The failure of emotional intelligence is seen as immature, irritable, or self-centered, but the root cause is a passive mind.

Related symptoms of a passive mind include the tendency to snap at others, slam doors, act upset without serious provocation, and generally exhibit self-involved behaviors. This emotional reactivity demonstrates an exaggerated need for self-gratification and lack of being in touch with the outside world. These behaviors push others away, and damage relationships. As Dr. Bradberry explains, "Expressing anger too much or at the wrong times desensitizes people to what you are feeling, making it hard for others to take you seriously."[193]

When we are passive-minded, we have little or no control, and therefore we reflexively express any negativity we may be feeling at the moment. Again, we are pushed around by external influences instead of taking command of the moment. "If you typically yell when you are feeling angry, for example, you have to learn to choose an alternative reaction."[194]

Self-gratifying anger behavior increases when the culture condones it. Screen culture produces this behavior and then reinforces it. The tendency to lose self control increases by time, and by each new generation, growing up with ever increasing screen-centric lifestyles. There is a huge gap in Emotional Intelligence (EQ) between the generations. Generation Y (bn. late 1980s–90s) are much more prone to fly off the handle when things don't go their way.[195]

Dr. Bradberry sums it up nicely: "One of the huge fallacies our culture has embraced is that feeling something is the same as acting on that feeling, and that's just wrong, because there's this little thing called self-control. Whether it's helping out a co-worker when you're in a crunch to meet your own deadline or continuing to be pleasant with someone who is failing to return the favor, being considerate often means not acting on what you feel."[196] "If you grow up in a culture where emotional outbursts and careless self-gratification are not only discouraged but are also considered personally shameful, such an upbringing is going to affect the way you manage yourself and others."[197]

Non-screen lifestyles produce more active self-management. Active-minded emotional intelligence means taking command of our moods in a more responsible fashion. "Emotionally intelligent people place high value on their relationships, which means they treat everyone with respect, regardless of the kind of mood they're in."[198]

Anger happens, but we can choose to override the passive reflex by processing the negative energy, to our own benefit. "Those who use the right tools and strategies for harnessing their emotions put themselves in a position to prosper."[199]

There is a significant "subjective-versus-objective" component to emotional intelligence. The self-gratifying reflex is symptomatic of being excessively subjective. It leads to being controlled by emotions with negative consequences. Consciously shifting to a more objective way of processing helps break this cycle of helplessness. "Your objectivity would allow you to step out from under the control of your emotions and know exactly what needed to be done to create a positive outcome."[200]

We can take command of the moment, and transform negative emotion into a different kind of energy. "While it's impossible not to feel your emotions, it's completely under your power to manage them effectively and to keep yourself in control of them. When you let your emotions overtake your ability to think clearly, it's easy to lose your resolve."[201]

By being more objective, we also gain clearer insight into self-improvement opportunities. For example, we are better equipped to benefit from criticism, by taking it thoughtfully, instead of being offended or reacting resentfully to criticism. Emotionally intelligent command of the moment includes a balanced response to criticism. For example, in an article about influential people, one characteristic is how they take criticism. When criticized, they "don't react immediately and emotionally. They wait. They think. And then they deliver an appropriate response. [They] know how important relationships are, and they won't let an emotional overreaction harm theirs. They also know that emotions are contagious, and overreacting has a negative influence on everyone around them." Similarly, they "do not react emotionally and defensively to dissenting opinions—they welcome them. They're humble enough to know that they don't know everything and that someone else might see something they missed. And if that person is right, they embrace the idea wholeheartedly because they care more about the end result than being right."[202]

Active minded people are open to criticism, open to opposing views from people they dislike, objective in their response to new information, not concerned about "being right," and not defensive. Greater emotional development allows more genuine openness to criticism and opposing viewpoints. It also allows stronger character-building and more advanced personal development.

Active-minded lifestyles lead to both stronger and more genuine personalities. "Genuine people have a strong enough sense of self that they don't go around seeing offense that isn't there. If somebody criticizes one of their ideas, they don't treat this as a personal attack. There's no need for them to…feel insulted…. They're able to objectively evaluate negative and constructive feedback, accept what works, put it into practice, and leave the rest of it behind without developing hard feelings."[203]

Objectivity is the key. Whether my mood is good or bad, being aware that it's just a mood, retaining an objective view of what I am going through, gives me better command, judgment, freedom, and success. As concentration-camp survivor Victor Frankl said: "Between stimulus and response there is a space. In that space is our power to choose our response. In our response lies our growth and our freedom."[204]

"Victor Frankl was not only a concentration camp survivor during the Holocaust, but also someone who went on to help others find goodness and meaning in life. He was a man from whom we can

67

learn something about what it means to be human and how to be our best—sometimes in spite of our inclinations."[205]

This is the hallmark of an active mind—it overrides weaker passive emotional reactions. It is another ingredient in a higher caliber lifestyle. It is the kind of higher functioning that is another casualty of a screen-centric lifestyle.

Passive Minds and Violence

Don't confuse a passive mind with nonviolence. Violent crime is the province of passive minds. A passive mind is undisciplined. It bottles up stress, frustration, oppressed feelings, and unmanaged anger, which produce the most erratic outbursts. The passive mind does not plan for the future, but waits for a pain-impulse to force an immediate-gratification action, such as hunger or drug-craving, or sudden eruption of pent up frustrations. The impulse on a passive mind triggers the emotionally undeveloped reflex of violence, which has no reasonable or apparent provocation.

Recent studies have shown that unprovoked or out-of-proportion violence against others becomes more likely in the absence of healthy social time with others. Life has been mostly one of isolation from people, therefore there is no empathy or caring for others.[206] It has also been shown that minds made passive by watching too much TV carry more aggression and are more likely to commit crimes.[207]

Since passive screen-centric lifestyles lead to more aggression and crime, the reverse is obviously true: less passive screentime produces less erratic aggression and less crime.

It is important to note here, that the violent tendency is from screentime, of any kind, regardless of programming. When we fail to recognize that the problem is with the screen, instead of what's on the screen, we fall into the same rut of denial. We fail to confront the root cause of many of our social ills today.

Fighting is Good for Boys

Violence is the disease, fighting is the cure. Does that sound counterintuitive? Let's follow the breadcrumbs and see how we get to that statement.

An additional factor is that society has become more feminine in recent generations.[208] In addition, men today are significantly weaker physically than men in the past.[209] This assertion might irk some men to hear it, but it is the least controversial statement so far. We shouldn't need a study to see the fact. Daily activities of men in both job life and personal life require much less physical exertion. It's also true that men sit around and watch TV, which they didn't do in the past.

But what does the femininization of society have to do with fighting being good for boys? One of the outcomes of weaker men and a more feminine society is an increasingly negative view of fighting.

Throughout history, boys by the age of 10 would have been in many fights and wrestling matches, on the playground, in the neighborhood, wherever kids go. It happens less nowadays, partly because society has become more feminine[210], which can have a damping effect on some traditional male behaviors such as fighting.[211]

A study reported by the *Child Trends Databank* found that "The share of students in grades 9 through 12 who had been in at least one physical fight in the past year declined from 43 percent in 1991 to 33 percent in 2001. The proportion remained steady until 2011, between 32 and 36 percent. However, between 2011 and 2015 the proportion decreased markedly, from 33 to 23 percent."[212]

The years 2011 to 2015 correspond to the years that smartphones became universal. We increased from too much screentime up to 2011, to way too much screentime by 2015.

With continuous screen-device-time, natural behaviors such as boys fighting became suppressed even more than in previous years. There is at least a coinciding pattern that males' screentime parallels the pattern of males becoming more feminine, with natural male behaviors being suppressed in an unhealthy way.

A study reported in *The Oxford Handbook of the Development of Play* found that the subtleties of fighting are typically male specific. Showing videos of healthy fighting versus serious or vicious fighting, men could tell the difference, women who grew up with brothers could tell the difference. But women who hadn't grown up with brothers could not tell the difference—they mostly thought all of the videos equally involved serious fighting.[213] Overall feminine socialization and behavioral expectations means healthy fighting is increasingly viewed the same as unhealthy or vicious fighting, seen as indistinguishable and wrong. "Adults, especially women who aren't personally familiar with rough play often try to stop rough-housing because they don't want anyone to get hurt. But research tells us that, overall, rough play turns into a real fight only about 1% of the time among elementary school boys."[214]

Unfortunately, boys who grow up to be adults without this natural formative interaction will grow up unhealthy, with less emotional intelligence, less mature self-governance, ill-equipped for healthy confrontation during conflicts in later life, developing less camaraderie and less connection to others. Men evolved to need this activity in order to develop normally. Screentime is robbing men and society at large from this area of healthy socialization.

For example, an Iowa State University study found that TV viewing is linked to ADHD[215], and in an ADHD study, "Intriguing research by neuroscientist Jaak Panksepp shows that giving young, hyperactive lots of opportunity to do play fighting helps them learn to inhibit their behavior."[216] Combine this with the proven correlation between TV viewing and criminal behavior[217], and we begin to see a troubling picture of unhealthy suppression of fighting, which undermines mental stability, and increases risk of criminal behavior.

The conclusion seems clear enough. If we reduce boys' screentime, and let their natural instincts take their course, we are all better off. Conversely, a continuation of today's screen-isolation behaviors will lead to more aggression, criminal behaviors, and out-of-proportion violence.[218] As in a multitude of mental-health issues we have seen up to now, the first step is to acknowledge the destructiveness of our screen-centric lifestyles.

PART II:
Better Ways

CHAPTER 6: THE PSYCHOLOGY OF TRUE SELF WORTH VERSUS FALSE SELF ESTEEM

The healthy response to mistakes is to accept responsibility. Blaming circumstances and other people surrenders your self-worth and your future to the control of others. As clinical psychologist Travis Bradberry explains, "Here's the worst thing about feeling sorry for yourself, other than it being annoying, of course: it shifts your locus of control outside yourself. Feeling sorry for yourself is, in essence, declaring that you're a helpless victim of circumstance. Emotionally intelligent people never feel sorry for themselves because that would mean giving up their power."[219]

Our choices create our journey and determine our destination. It's not society's fault, it's not the economy's fault, it's not my parents' fault, it's not my kids' fault, it's not my circumstance's fault. It's my fault. A sincere, genuine individual does not point at other people, or at circumstances, but looks in the mirror and says "I did this." Mean it and understand it. The passive mind's response to failure will be exaggerated rather than sincere and accurate.

Two typical extremes of the passive mind are
1. "I'm great and nothing was my fault," the inflated-ego syndrome

   or the other extreme,
2. "I'm a no-good failure, there's no use trying," the self-loathing syndrome.

Both are lazy cover-ups.

It takes energy to change or improve. Passivity leads to do-nothing responses: "I'm great as I am, no change needed"; or, "I'm a total failure, no change possible, no use trying."

In both extreme-passive cases, there is no hope for fixing what's broken, because there's no accurate appraisal of what's broken.

Even the "total-failure" case does not recognize what's broken accurately. It merely hides a fixable flaw behind a perversely exaggerated cloud of grotesque self-loathing. As *The Motivation*

Myth author Jeff Haden notes, "Hide from your weaknesses, and you'll always be weak. Accept your weaknesses and work to improve them, and you'll eventually be stronger—and more motivated to keep improving."[220]

The two dishonest tactics—inflated-ego and self-loathing—let the passive mind dodge accountability for mistakes. "If you are someone who thinks either *it's all my fault* or *it's all their fault* you are wrong most of the time."[221]

- Inflated-ego: "I did everything right. My problems are not my fault. Look at the bad luck I had to deal with, look at what happened that I couldn't control, look at what they did that made it harder to avoid, look everywhere else, but don't look at me."
- Self-loathing: "I'm such a mess, I can't do anything right. Why should I even try, I can't change who I am! I'm a failure and I might as well accept it."

These two dishonest tactics are also lazy tactics. An inactive approach to problems follows from an inactive mind, which follows from too much screentime.

The only way to grow out of these passive-avoidance tactics is to acknowledge responsibility, to sincerely accept accountability, to respond with positive determination: "Emotionally intelligent people know that success lies in their ability to rise in the face of failure."[222] By following the path of responsible accountability, we learn that "If I do good things, good things happen, if I do bad things, bad things happen, and if I do nothing, nothing happens."[223]

The result is amazing: better response, better results, better self-worth. "By holding yourself accountable, even when making excuses is an option, you show that you care about results more than your image or ego."[224]

False Positive Self-Esteem

Our society's emphasis on a positive self-esteem for its own sake conflicts with true self-worth. We can't force-fit "high self-esteem" onto someone who hasn't earned it, any more than we can force-fit claims of "high quality" onto poor craftsmanship.

One of the worst, and most typical, forms this takes is the self-proclaimed declaration of greatness. This is when people announce grand plans to do something admirable. Author Jeff Haden provides a great example: a friend in a restaurant says he plans to hike the entire 2,200-mile Appalachian Trail. He talks about equipment he's buying, maps he's collecting, how it will take six months of hard work. Surrounded by amazed admiration, the friend is already basking in the glow of the accomplishment. In fact, he is in an air-conditioned restaurant and will later drive home to his comfy bed.[225]

But will he follow through? Science says, probably not. People who announce great plans are much less likely to translate it to action.[226] He will not walk the talk, literally. He will never set foot on the Appalachian Trail. He doesn't have to because he already received the high from being admired: "this gives the individual a premature sense of possessing the aspired-to identity."[227] He is viewed as a great hiker, or at least he feels he is viewed as such.

Conversely, people who quietly plan are the doers who are much more likely to achieve.

In many ways, self-aggrandizement is an indulgence that is a temporary fix to an unproductive life. But the subconscious mind is not fooled by the trick of artificial high self-esteem.

The trick involves denial of one's true self, to avoid uncomfortable challenges such as accountability and work. As clinical psychologist Dr. Bradberry explains, "The biggest obstacle to increasing your self-awareness is the tendency to avoid the discomfort that comes from seeing yourself as you really are. Things you do not think about … can sting when they surface. Avoiding this pain creates problems, because it is merely a short-term fix. You'll never be able to manage yourself effectively if you ignore what you need to do to change."[228]

Authentic self-worth comes from hard work, endurance, character, integrity, and responsibility, while achieving goals. Apply that kind of discipline, and we naturally produce a positive self-image. We don't have to claim it or promote it. We don't have to trick ourselves into it. We accomplish self-worth organically by our actions and our track record.

Conversely, self-conscious emphasis on high self-esteem causes low self-esteem. It is especially damaging to children. For example, artificially promoting high self-esteem by being overly protective undermines healthy development and ownership of actions. "Unfortunately, without this sense of ownership, children are thoroughly unprepared for the adulthood because in the real world our actions do have consequences."[229]

Exaggerated praise and over-protectiveness produce people who have to beg for attention to feel good. Self-esteem depends on one's ego being stroked by others. "People who are always begging for attention are needy. They rely on that attention from other people to form their self-identity."[230] The result is a fragile and false self-esteem that easily crumbles. Needy self-esteem is a trap of vulnerability and insincerity.

Genuine self-worth allows for a more genuine personality: "They aren't driven by ego. … They simply do what needs to be done without saying, 'Hey, look at me!'"[231] With a more substantial self-esteem gained by effort and productivity, we don't need accolades in order to feel good. But the more time wasted in passive screentime, the less equipped we are to achieve this quiet road to genuine self-worth.

Dr. Bradberry brings it into perspective: "While it's impossible to turn off your reactions to what others think of you, you don't have to compare yourself with others, and you can always take people's opinions with a grain of salt. That way, no matter what other people are thinking or doing, your self-worth comes from within."[232] Work and achievement feed a virtuous cycle of inner strength and value.

Career Shock

When a parent or a mentor says, "you can be whatever you want to be," there's an opportunity to ask questions, and talk about what it takes to achieve something in the real world. Too often on TV shows and in commercials, "you can be whatever you want to be," becomes a promise in a vacuum. The message implants the passive version of the dream into our consciousness: If I imagine it, it will just happen. It becomes a false hope without the two-way conversation needed to put dreams and reality into perspective.

As screentime replaces realtime over the formative years, the gap widens between screen-fed false hopes and real-world requirements. After college, when we start looking for a job, we experience a traumatic shock. Screen-life left us unaware, unprepared, and ill-equipped. The jarring incongruity between pre-career fantasies and the real job market has grown increasingly common over recent generations.

College Recruiter explains it this way: "Despite all of your job hunting efforts, however, you find that getting your dream job is not as easy as you hoped … in order to get into the job market, you need to take a good look at all of the available choices, adjust your preferences to 'fit in,' and give it your best shot. While it may come as a shock to you, many graduates end up never working in their major. In fact, the majority of graduates don't get to use their degrees at all, and most feel that they are forced to follow a different direction."[233]

While creativity can help advance a career, jobs themselves are typically not very creative. "You'll probably have to pursue your passions during your off-time."[234]

As a result of the screen-fed career fantasy, we graduate from college assuming that a comfortable position will just happen; instead of having to submit hundreds of applications to score a subsistence-level job that is not fun at all. Years of hopeful anticipation evaporate into hopeless demoralization. The letdown follows from an upbringing without strict, painful discipline—the result is increasingly indicated by a screen-centric childhood.

The opposite follows from an active nonscreen childhood, where the tools of initiative and emotional maturity equip us with a make-the-most-of-it approach.

Clinical psychologist and author Dr. Travis Bradberry reinforces this idea, "Emotionally intelligent people believe that the world is a meritocracy and that the only things that they deserve are those that they earn. People who lack EQ often feel entitled. They think that the world owes them something. Again, it's about locus of control. Emotionally intelligent people know that they alone are responsible for their successes or failures."[235]

We expect to work hard, and feel grateful for any chance to get a foot in the door to prove ourselves. We are better-prepared for hardship and delayed gratification, such as putting in extra hours at night and on weekends for no extra pay or recognition. This personal investment emphasizes personal responsibility for career growth. Recognition and promotions may come later after years of proof. As *The Motivation Myth* author Jeff Haden reminds us, "While you ultimately may want to prove that you have the potential to hold higher-level positions, your immediate goal is to be the best in your company at what you *currently* do."[236]

Achievers will spend their own time and money to gain professional knowledge, to earn the advantage, knowing that rewards come after years of high performance. *Motivation* author Haden continues this idea: "They prepare. They train. They constantly experiment and adapt and refine, refine, refine. Highly accomplished people gain superior skills not by bursting through the envelope but by approaching and then slowly and incrementally expanding the boundaries of that envelope."[237]

The ability to thrive amid the tough entry-level reality generates a career path that grows steadily after repeated accomplishment. Again from Jeff Haden, "Don't be fooled by the work-life-balance fluff. Tremendous effort and dedication are required…. The only way is the hard way."[238]

From the trenches to the top, hard work builds gratifying self-worth and lifelong fulfillment. When you begin to love the struggle as much the achievement, you've crossed the line into a successful mentality. It's a mentality that leads to meaningful progress.

Builders versus Bellyachers

There are lots of kinds of people in the world. This section looks at two distinct types: builders and bellyachers.

A builder is someone with initiative who contributes productivity and positive energy to others. A bellyacher is a procrastinator who is unproductive and drains energy from others.

Initiative makes people shine. Procrastination makes people dull. Lesson learned: Start each day by eating the frog.[239] That is, "I commit to take care of the worst thing on my plate first every day." Delaying the unpleasant is a telltale sign of the bellyacher, who spends the day, the month, the lifetime, dreading a mounting avalanche of unpleasant tasks.

The result of delaying work is the piling up of work. Anxiety mounts, stress increases, direct or indirect punishments and penalties ensue. Helpless frustration is often vented at other people, which builds nothing, except a reputation for incompetence. Dr. Bradberry puts it into perspective: "Every moment spent dreading the task subtracts time and energy from actually getting it done. People that learn to habitually make the tough calls stand out like flamingos in a flock of seagulls."[240]

Builders spend every day productively. And they test limits. As author Jeff Haden aptly describes it, "We all have a little voice inside that says, 'I've done enough' or 'I'm exhausted. I just can't do more.' But that little voice lies. We can always do more. Stopping is a choice." A builder's typical day is what Haden calls an Extreme Productivity Day (EPD).[241] It isn't easy, but builders make it every day. Soon it becomes second nature.

Making mistakes is another differentiator between builders and bellyachers. Everyone makes mistakes. Builders are deeply troubled by mistakes, but they don't waste energy and other people's time making excuses or complaining about it. Another Bradberry perspective: "You have to make mistakes, look like an idiot, and try again—without even flinching."[242]

Complaining gets in the way of conquering. If it doesn't go well at first, builders solve problems, recover from failures, and improve. Per Bradberry, "When hard times hit, people with mental strength suffer just as much as everyone else. The difference is that they understand that life's challenging moments offer valuable lessons. In the end, it's these tough lessons that build the strength you need to succeed."[243]

Bradberry delivers the appropriate ultimatum, "You always have two choices when things begin to get tough: you can either overcome an obstacle and grow in the process or let it beat you. Humans are creatures of habit. If you quit when things get tough, it gets that much easier to quit the next time. On the other hand, if you force yourself to push through a challenge, the strength begins to grow in you."[244]

Builders focus on trying harder, determined to move forward with a purpose. They see the mountaintop and do not hesitate to take the first step. A recent study at the College of William and Mary found that the most successful entrepreneurs can't even imagine failure (even if they've had past failures), and pay no attention to naysayers.[245] Both success and failure teach lessons. Builders learn from both and keep growing.

Bellyachers do very little, but expect very much, and complain that the world isn't fair. Bradberry pulls no punches: "Negative people are bad news because they wallow in their problems and fail to focus on solutions. They want people to join their pity party so that they can feel better about themselves."[246] They stand around in a field of possibilities all their lives, kicking the dirt around, but never building anything. Their world becomes a land of broken dreams and failed potential. Bellyachers will never live life to the fullest, never put the most into it, and never get the most out of it.

Delayed Gratification

Like virtually everyone from the beginning of human history until the mid-twentieth century, builders understand delayed gratification. As *Motivation* author Jeff Haden notes, "Successful people are great at delaying gratification. Successful people are great at withstanding temptation."[247]

The well-known Stanford experiment of a child and a marshmallow tell us all we need to know about the importance of delayed gratification: "There was a famous Stanford experiment in which an administrator left a child in a room with a marshmallow for 15 minutes. Before leaving, the experimenter told the child that she was welcome to eat it, but if she waited until he returned without eating it, she would get a second marshmallow. The children that were able to wait until the experimenter returned experienced better outcomes in life, including higher SAT scores, greater career success, and even lower body mass indexes."[248]

Anyone can have dreams. Anyone can envision greatness. But success comes only from taking the first tiny steps, knowing that years and miles of lonely discipline must come first. Haden is great at condensing the point to its essential ingredient: "We all *say* we want to achieve things, but we don't really want to achieve them unless we are willing to take the necessary steps to achieve what we say we want."[249]

- The failed person cannot take the first of 10,000 steps, because it seems too long and too hard and too far away. The failed person cannot imagine thriving until the goal "happens."
- Mode of Travel Is the End in Itself: The successful person thrives on the process, on every step of the way during years and miles of lonely pain. The goal remains in the back of the mind, but satisfaction continuously fills the mind and heart from the struggle itself.
- Screen-centered behaviors indicate failed outcomes.
- Non-screen-centered behaviors indicate successful outcomes.

The key takeaway on this topic is simple: "Delayed gratification is always better gratification."[250]

Complete Perfectionists

Complete Perfectionists (as opposed to Compartmentalized Perfectionists discussed in a later section) are builders who take building to the highest level. They are the exceptional ones with extraordinary determination. Every excellence achieved is merely another unsatisfactory starting point upon which to improve.

These perfectionists have a heightened sense of order and exactitude from the biggest big picture to the tiniest detail. Their antennae register the risk of error with devastating sensitivity. When they make a mistake, they don't flinch or break stride. They take the immediate next step to recover from it.

Fretting over a mistake is impossible for perfectionists. They develop ways to move forward rapidly after a mistake without a blink. They get it right and keep doing better. They plow ahead despite opposition, failure, and danger. They have extraordinary emotional intelligence in areas of achievement. "Emotionally intelligent people persevere. They don't give up in the face of failure, and they don't give up because they're tired or uncomfortable. They're focused on their goals, not on momentary feelings, and that keeps them going even when things are hard."[251] This could be said of any builder or active-minded person, but perfectionists push it harder.

Perfectionists take seriously the importance of poise and fortitude under duress. Their sacred duty is to make difficult work look easy. The "make-it-look-easy" theme is common when talking about people who excelled in their careers and soared in their disciplines. To cite a couple of refreshing examples:

- Dick Van Dyke said of Stan Laurel (of the *Laurel and Hardy* comedy duo), about the artistic effort in his work: "Stan took care to hide it, to conceal the hours of hard creative work that went into his movies. He didn't want you to see that—he just wanted you to laugh, and you did!"[252]
- From a *biography.com* sketch of Fred Astaire: "Fred Astaire revolutionized the movie musical with his elegant and seemingly effortless dance style. He may have made dancing look easy, but he was a well-known perfectionist, and his work was the product of endless hours of practice."[253]

These examples express the idea of perfectionism, but more important, they can serve as inspiration for others.

Perfectionist versus Frustrationist

A phony perfectionist wants everything to be perfect now, without real effort. Phony perfectionists complain about imperfections and then do nothing to overcome them. They are frustrated by a mistake, but don't work to correct it.

If I say, "I get frustrated a lot because I'm such a perfectionist," I am merely a frustrationist. Perfectionists don't dwell on frustration, and certainly don't mention it to others.

Envying someone else's achievements betrays frustration, which comes from a passive mind. A frustrationist wants others to do worse, "so I look better."

This passive-comparison tendency is linked to the artificial-self-esteem tendency—to artificially elevate one's own self-esteem without the painful work of earning it. Self-image goes up when others go down. The trick of comparison-with-others is a disingenuous substitute for the genuine person's healthy habit of comparing self with self. It belies a screen-life bereft of emotional development.

True perfectionists do not compare self to others, but compare self "as is" to self "as could be." The perfect tendency is to push the boundary of my own higher potential. This kind of emotional intelligence produces healthy motivation, which fuels genuine confidence. Genuine people insist on healthy process.

Dr. Travis Bradberry frames the idea nicely: "Emotionally intelligent people understand that the happiness and success of others doesn't take away from their own, so jealousy and envy aren't an issue for them. They see success as being in unlimited supply, so they can celebrate others' successes."[254] A perfectionist values genuineness above all. Genuine people "want you to do well more than anything else because they're … confident enough to never worry that your success might make them look bad. In fact, they believe that your success is their success."[255]

Perfectionists share a deep desire for all things in life to excel and draw closer to perfection—in oneself, in others, and in all things. Perfectionists are also too generous to wish failure upon others.

Being considerate is a virtue in itself, and that is another piece of the perfectionist's puzzle.

Another Bradberry gem: "Many people approach life as a zero-sum game. They think that somebody has to win and somebody else has to lose. Considerate people, on the other hand, try to find a way for everybody to win. That's not always possible, but it's their goal."[256]

Real perfectionists want a world filled with the highest caliber people, achieving great successes, raising the bar every day. Every step in that direction is celebrated quietly, while striving to do better.

The Spectrum

Being a perfectionist takes the normal healthy ways of living as a builder, and increases the energy beyond the limits of most people.

Everyone falls somewhere in the spectrum between "no perfectionist characteristics" and a "complete perfectionist." Most people tend towards one end or the other—builders on the perfectionist end, bellyachers on the other end. Everyone is somewhere in between because, after all, nobody's perfect. The lesson is to fight the good fight towards improvement.

Before the mid-twentieth century, the population tended towards the builder end of the spectrum. Because of screen-based mental deterioration and physical decline, the trend is now towards the bellyacher end.

Compartmentalized Perfectionism

What about the Vincent van Goghs of this world, who are widely viewed as perfectionists in their specialty, but whose lives are a disaster in other areas? These are cases of "compartmentalized perfectionism": geniuses who focus in their expertise, such as painting, but are far from perfect in other areas.

Vincent van Gogh is an extreme case in point. He was in and out of an asylum, and ultimately committed suicide. But he created over 2,000 paintings and drawings from 1880 to 1890. About 900 of those were fully realized paintings. That's at least seven paintings and nine drawings per month, every month, for ten years.[257] At today's values, van Gogh would be making about $10 million per month. He didn't get a penny.

He painted because he was a perfect artist—he couldn't not paint. He suffered in a quiet storm of passion to the death. The classic warning "Don't try this at home" applies. The compartmentalized perfectionist is romanticized and sometimes might benefit posterity is some way. But such opposing extremes in one person is not a recipe for healthy living.

CHAPTER 7: THOUGHTFULNESS AND WISDOM

Thoughtful can mean both "kind" and "thinking." Historically the two were closely related. It was the sign of a thinking person to act with appreciation and gratitude, to practice good manners, to show sincere courtesy towards others. It is obvious that courtesy has diminished markedly in our society. As clinical psychologist and *Emotional Intelligence 2.0* author Travis Bradberry notes, "With the decline of good manners, there are fewer expressions of appreciation."[258]

Courtesy evolved as a vital aspect of wisdom, because thinking people understood the far-reaching personal and social benefits of a thoughtful and courteous population. Thinking through to the logical conclusion, if courtesy and thoughtfulness were the rule rather than the exception throughout the population, we would enjoy being around other people more. There would be less stress and more camaraderie.

Notice the emphasis is on the positive effect on everyone, on *other people*. Dr. Bradberry explains, "A lot of people have come to believe that not only are manners unnecessary, they're undesirable because they're fake. These people think that being polite means you're acting in a way that doesn't reflect how you actually feel, but they've got it backwards. 'Minding your manners' is all about focusing on how the other person feels, not on how *you* feel. It's consciously acting in a way that puts other people at ease and makes them feel comfortable."[259]

Discourtesy is a self-indulgent trait symptomatic of a screen-centric life. The symptoms arise from both the mental-disengagement and the isolation caused by screentime.

Courtesy, on the other hand, would improve everyday life for everyone. We would look forward to simple activities like buying groceries, driving to work, stopping at the bank, shopping for clothes; because those activities involve seeing people, who would be a pleasure to interact with as a rule. This healthier and happier life is a fact of brain chemistry and the positive feelings we receive from positive encounters.

We would be more willing to take our free-time activities out around other people: going to parks, walking in the neighborhood, sitting outside saying hello to neighbors passing by, walking downtown, visiting the library, going to outdoor markets, participating in community events. Courtesy and camaraderie shine a brighter light on every social activity.

It almost seems like a dream of yesteryear to many, the ideas of enjoying meeting people, enjoying talking with "strangers" out in public every day. It was normal and common for thousands of years.

We can still learn from the 1340s cleric who said of Paradise, "There one learns to live well in wisdom and courtesy, for no villainy enters there."[260] It reminds us of the vital connection between wisdom and courtesy, and how much screenlife has made us forget. Who would not rather see a restoration of that connection? Why wouldn't we want to restore a sense of community, neighborliness, enjoying each other's company?

Clinical psychologist Travis Bradberry summarizes the practical benefits: "Being considerate is good for your mental and physical health, your career, and everyone around you."[261] Screentime remains our primary obstacle.

Listen to Communicate

There are a lot of ways to communicate. The best way is to listen. We can tell by the response when someone was not really listening. They reply with something that is off topic or incongruent. They ask a question that was just explained. Or they just ask us to repeat the whole thing because they "didn't catch it." Often the reply switches the focus over to the other person—the listener is sending a message: "Whatever you said, it's more interesting if we make it about me."

Most of us have experienced this, and we probably felt disappointment from a distracted or self-centered listener. In these cases, there is a subtle but real message of disrespect towards the speaker. As clinical psychologist Dr. Bradberry notes, "The biggest mistake people make when it comes to listening is they're so focused on what they're going to say next or how what the other person is saying is going to affect them that they fail to hear what's being said."[262]

It's worse when we let an electronic device blatantly divide our attention. As Dr. Bradberry notes, "Nothing will turn someone off to you like a mid-conversation text message or even a quick glance at your phone. When you commit to a conversation, focus all of your energy on the conversation."[263]

Conversely, it is rewarding and refreshing when a listener responds with an intelligent question that demonstrates attentiveness. Dr. Bradberry encourages this kind of attentiveness: "When someone is talking to you, stop everything else and listen fully until the other person is finished speaking ... pick up on the cues the other person sends, and really hear what he or she is saying."[264]

Aside from the courtesy element, there is a self-improvement element. People who learn the most, listen the best. As Hemingway noted, "I like to listen. I have learned a great deal from listening carefully. Most people never listen."[265]

Happy Minded

An active mind makes us happier. The active-happy correlation is a strong one that has been well known for hundreds of years. As British Prime Minister Benjamin Disraeli said in 1884, "Action may not always bring happiness; but there is no happiness without action."[266] That goes for both mental and physical action. Aristotle puts it simply: "Happiness is a state of activity."[267] By implication, watching videos is a state of unhappiness. In fact, as a study reported in the *Journal of Economic Psychology* makes clear, TV viewing decreases life satisfaction, and increases anxiety.[268]

What are happy people like? The people who seem happiest, seem happiest no matter what happens to them, good or bad. As noted in by experts in this area Drs. Jean Greaves and Travis Bradberry, "Even when you can't do or say anything to change a difficult situation, you always have a say in your perspective of what's happening, which ultimately influences your feeling about it."[269]

For an unhappy-passive mind, a little trouble generates a lot of bitterness. A little success breeds a lot of gloating and exaggerated celebration. An unhappy-passive mind handles both success and failure poorly, and learns from neither.

For a happy-active mind, a lot of trouble does not cause bitterness, but increases fortitude. Success breeds no gloating, but more humility and perseverance to succeed more. Active-happy-minded people handle both success and failure with grace and learn from both.

Active minds are happier because they process incoming data more effectively. That in itself leads to healthier brain-chemical reactions. It is so simple, it becomes a matter of statistical predictability. From a 2012 *Ted Talk*: "if I know everything about your external world, I can only predict 10 percent of your long-term happiness. 90 percent of your long-term happiness is predicted not by the external world, but by the way your brain processes the world."[270]

Active minds are less dependent on external circumstances for happiness. The brain naturally generates happiness as a mode of travel through life. A Passive mind doesn't process life in a healthy way, so it inevitably views happiness as an object to obtain. Grasping for happiness like an object is the most famous road to frustration and misery.

Wise people have known that happiness is a mode of travel, and a way of processing, since the beginning of time. Founding Mother Martha Washington, for example, said "for I have also learnt, from experience, that the greater part of our happiness or misery depends upon our dispositions, and not upon our circumstances. We carry the seeds of the one or the other about with us, in our minds, wheresoever we go."[271]

Viktor Frankl was a concentration-camp survivor during the WWII Holocaust. There is perhaps no better authority on the choice of how we respond to circumstances. Frankl points out that "people often react without thinking. We frequently don't choose our behaviors so much as just act them out. But [Frankl] observes that we don't need to accept such reflexive reactions. Instead, we can learn to notice that there is a 'space' before we react. He suggests that we can grow and change and be different if we can learn to recognize, increase, and make use of this 'space.' With such awareness, we can find freedom from the dictates of both external and internal pressures. And with that, we can find inner happiness."[272]

A passive-screen-entertainment lifestyle makes it harder to process experiences in a healthy way. When effort and activity replace screentime, we have a chance to heal our brain's mode of processing . Then we have a chance to shift from frustrated grasping, to successful living. Franklin Delano Roosevelt offers a last thought on this topic: "Happiness lies in the joy of achievement and the thrill of creative effort."[273]

Intuition and Decisions

Following only emotions usually leads to unhappiness. Purely practical considerations can also lead to unhappiness. Emotional and practical considerations are important, but not enough alone. The critical ingredient to align person with path is intuition.

Intuition is a deep awareness of both external surroundings and internal self. It is a more complex faculty that includes both emotional and rational awareness. It may be a prediction, an idea that a friend has a problem, a sense of "knowing" that we'll like someone when we first meet them, a decision we have to make at work when there is not adequate information, "knowing" which way to turn at an unfamiliar intersection, a decision about a vacation, a sense that we will like this job but not that one, an insight in a conversation, studying a new subject, a decision on buying a house, and countless other situations. Intuition is, in a word, awareness.

As clinical psychologist Dr. Bradberry explains, "Awareness of yourself is not just knowing that you are a morning person instead of a night owl. It's deeper than that. Getting to know yourself inside and out is a continuous journey of peeling back the layers of the onion and becoming more and more comfortable with what is in the middle—the true essence of you."[274]

Often we may see the right path or the right decision for us, but we give in to outside pressures and lose confidence. Perhaps the most important criterion for our own fulfillment, after making the best possible decision, is to trust it. Don't give in to other people's doubts and criticisms. Awareness means mental strength that values our own intuitive thinking: "People with mental strength believe in themselves no matter what, and they stay the course."[275] Turn to intuition more than mere emotions and mere practicality for guidance, then trust it.

Intuition doesn't magically happen out of the blue. It takes all that time we spent in front of TV and then some. For example, following a momentary gut feeling and just going with it, without reflection, can be just as misguided as ignoring intuition altogether. Intuition, or deeper awareness, comes from spending time reflecting on facts and data that make up our lives. Rapid surface calculations of experiences and options do not return intuitive insights. Time, focus, perception, and reflection are integral ingredients. These cognitive processes are undermined by screentime. Cognitive reflection helps us exercise and refine our intuition to serve us better.[276] Practicing and cultivating intuitive judgment with cognitive reflection are associated with higher functioning minds, which does not come from a screen-centric lifestyle.

The more important the decision is, the more important intuition becomes. Some life-changing, life-long choices are made while we're very young; career and marriage, for example. Childhood screentime robs us of intuitive decision-making skills that become critical in young adulthood. Failing that development, a lot more bad choices and regrets will follow.

The Aged and the Handmade

One way to deepen life experience is to find some good old-fashioned hidden beauty in the asymmetrical, individual, authentic, quirky, natural characteristics of people and objects. This beauty elevates authenticity, behaving in natural ways, uniqueness of appearances, appreciating diversity of talents, valuing different styles of expression—the expressions of people and nature.

These older concepts of beauty have been largely forgotten in the current era of virtual reality, sparkling HD screens, laser-precision industry, and special effects. Older concepts of beauty require long attention spans, focused concentration, reflective patience, close observation in the natural, three-dimensional world. They do not occur on a screen.

This kind of beauty requires a minimalist sensibility that celebrates the imperfect, unique, understated, authentic qualities of people and things. It emphasizes characteristics that are not obvious. It might be the beauty of a crack in a table that brings back fond memories of an event thirty years ago, or an imperfection in someone's face that makes the person more attractive and interesting. Older concepts of beauty are the opposite of CGI and polish.

Another example might be the sparse beauty of a small home with a nonsymmetrical meticulous interior, a few well-made pieces of essential furniture, with very tasteful but very little decoration.

Authentic beauty shines in the marks of aging in a person, or the effects of the elements on weathered objects. It could be the character in an aged person's face and hands, or the glow of a 90-year-old man's understated smile playing off his weathered skin. It might be an old pair of faded, torn, and patched blue-jeans. The emphasis is authenticity, so a brand-new pair of pre-faded, or pre-torn blue-jeans off the shelf would be a mockery of this kind of beauty—the opposite of life expression. Faded, worn, torn clothes from the wearer's activity over the years becomes an expression of that individual.

Old-fashioned beauty is also found in hand-crafted products. Factory-output products generally have geometrically even and symmetrical designs. Conversely, handmade tables, chairs, carpets, cabins, clothes, blankets, pottery, and most anything else handmade, show the uneven results inevitable with different individuals. We see expressions of design, manually crafting, carving, coloring, building, weaving, sewing, molding, and assembling. These reflect the uniquely human act of creation.

This kind of expression and effort gives the final product a depth that embodies the human spirit, making useful objects that also lend substance to everyday activities. It adds another dimension of meaning to life that is largely absent today.

We came to expect symmetry and perfection of design during the industrial revolution's mechanical exactness and consistent output, and even more so with computer-aided design, laser precision, geometrical balance to within a millionth of a millimeter, and colors measured to the exact CMYK ratio. These changes also change our perception of beauty, and we forget what it used to mean.

Wise Elders: An Endangered Species

The cumulative passive screentime for the whole population for the past sixty years means millions of lost hours of engagement with other people, including our most precious resource: Elders.

The only way to circulate the life learnings of older people is to pass it down to younger people who keep it alive. Otherwise, nothing is preserved or built upon, so the wealth of knowledge fades into extinction.

TV in the 1950s and 1960s marked a new phase when screen-centric culture began cutting off that circulation of knowledge. Today's devices finish cutting it off, as our immersion in screens fully displaces the human connections required to sustain that circulation. Ironically, the smartphone is the gravestone that marks the dead body of wisdom that once circulated in the veins of humanity.

Wisdom survives and grows only when all of us work, play, and live together, when we maximize in-person interaction. That is the way wisdom circulates. Given our amount of screentime today, we cannot possibly retain the wisdom of past generations. We certainly are not adding to it.

As we—the unwise screen-centered people—grow older, we have much less to pass along to the next generation. Each generation diminishes, gradually ending near zero. We cannot miss what we never noticed. Generations of knowledge and wisdom die away unmourned and unnoticed.

To give us a happier ending, all we need to do is turn away from our passive screen lifestyle. If we stop watching screens, the recirculation of knowledge will take care of itself.

Historia Magistra Vitae Est

As we lay to rest our dead elders, philosophers, prophets, poets, and all of our ancestors, we lose our deepest springs of life, we lose golden insights by the thousands. We replace a rich culture with a screen culture that keeps us distracted and thoughtless.

As we flutter around screens like moths, we lose priceless treasures and gain nothing. To quote a dead elder, Cicero, "Historia magistra vitae est"—History is the teacher of life—and we have lost our history.[277]

We are left with an intellectually and creatively bankrupt culture that was once animated and vibrant with deep experience and expression. Instead of being mourned, our golden ancestry is typically deprecated, denied, resented, laughed at, or dismissed as irrelevant. That is our mocking tribute.

Screenlife makes us settle for less, without knowing it. We settle for less in our society, and in ourselves. The degradation of our soul as a people follows from surrendering our best selves. But we can reclaim our better selves, resuscitate the circulation of wisdom, and restore a vibrant culture by cutting out the screen. It really is that simple.

CHAPTER 8: EPILOGUE

Here is one important takeaway from this book:
1. Easy is empty, difficult is rewarding

Mistakes can produce two kinds of responses:
1. Negative response: "I'm only human (I accept the lesser me)"
2. Positive response: "I'm fully human (I demand a better me)"

Only Human versus Fully Human

When a passive mind meets a high standard, he says "Nobody can measure up to that, it's not human!"

When a bellyacher meets a builder, he says "We're not all Superman! He's not human!"

People justify a low-caliber lifestyle by saying "I'm only human!"

Being "only human" means being incompetent, unreliable, weak, and careless. It means that humans who try harder are not human because they try harder. This is the prevailing attitude in a screen culture of passive entertainment.

The truth is, however, achievement makes the more disciplined person live more fully. As *The Motivation Myth* author Jeff Haden bluntly puts it: "If I haven't convinced you that being a serial achiever is the best way to live a full, satisfying, and successful professional life and personal life ... well, there's no hope for you."[278] By being active, strong, creative, reliable, and competent, the disciplined person is more fully human.

A Different Kind of Smart

Intelligence as measured by typical assessments does not guarantee success or even make it more likely. A passion to persevere and improve has a stronger correlation to success, because it is an active-minded characteristic.

Standard measures of intelligence tell nothing of the quality of person—or quality of life—compared to the measure of an active mind versus passive mind. That is why Emotional Intelligence (EQ) is so much more important than IQ. There are two import practical differences between IQ and EQ, as described by *Emotional Intelligence 2.0* author and clinical psychologist Travis Bradberry:

1. IQ is an innate characteristic that cannot be increased; but EQ is a skillset and a discipline that we can choose to develop.[279]
2. EQ is a much stronger indicator of success than IQ.[280]

This is an amazing gift! The tools for success and happiness are within our control, if we want it badly enough. The first building block is to establish daily active-minded habits. The choice is ours to embrace.

- High EQ is the hallmark of the active mind.
- Low EQ is the hallmark of the passive mind.

Psychologist Angela Duckworth spent years studying what makes high achievers so successful. Her results provide us with useful advice that we can put into action:

> "It wasn't SAT scores. It wasn't IQ scores. It wasn't even a degree from a top-ranking business school that turned out to be the best predictor of success. 'It was this combination of passion and perseverance that made high achievers special,' Duckworth said. 'In a word, they had grit.' Being gritty, according to Duckworth, is the ability to persevere. It's about being unusually resilient and hardworking, so much so that you're willing to continue on in the face of difficulties, obstacles and even failures. It's about being constantly driven to improve. In addition to perseverance, being gritty is also about being passionate about something. For the highly successful, Duckworth found that the journey was just as important as the end result. 'Even if some of the things they had to do were boring, or frustrating, or even painful, they wouldn't dream of giving up. Their passion was enduring.'"[281]

The key to this story is having the passion to push through boring and painful work. Passion is not about joy. It's about pain.

In another study, "only 25 percent of job successes are predicted by IQ, 75 percent of job successes are predicted by your optimism levels, your social support and your ability to see stress as a challenge instead of as a threat."[282]

In another example, Jon Morrow, an all-around thinker who is well-known in the world of blogging, provides a good example of active-minded smarts trumping conventional IQ measurements, in two of his 2014 posts ("How to Be Smart in a World of Dumb Bloggers" and "On Gluttony, Selfishness, and Unleashing the Power Within").[283] His self-avowed average IQ by standard measures had no negative impact on his rise to the top in his business. His passion, dedication, and purposeful development resulted in success. "Each and every popular blogger I know spends at least three or four hours a day consuming new information. It's not just an idiosyncrasy. It's *required*."[284]

All of these studies and examples lead to one conclusion: The best kind of "smart" is active-minded Emotional Intelligence (EQ), away from passive screen stagnation.

TV Drains the Color Out of Life

People used to say the 1960s is when the world became more colorful (applying a metaphor of color-TV technology and colorful 1960s styles). But the truth is, because of color TV, the 1960s is when the color drained from the world, and faded to black-and-white. As TV changed from gray to color, we changed from color to gray.

Today we mourn the loss of strength, the loss of wisdom, the loss of discipline, the loss of inventiveness, the loss of initiative, the loss of camaraderie. Video consumption is like a pill that decays these areas, while temporarily stimulating pleasant sensations. Every video, every TV show, is another pill that we swallow.

The Myth of the Myth

Some people claim a book like this is inventing a mythology: The myth of a greater civilization that is now lost, a romantic notion of a stronger, smarter, nobler, more capable species that roamed the earth in the legendary past.

If only it was a myth, we could breathe a sigh of relief. Unfortunately, we now have an overwhelming abundance of scientifically irrefutable findings. They show consistently over the past forty years that screentime has damaged our mental functioning, mental health, emotional development, and physical health.

With findings that are so consistent globally and across generations, we have a responsibility to respond in a fully human way, which shows character and integrity, not to mention hope for tomorrow.

We have to make a choice. Continuing our status quo screen-centric lifestyles is itself a choice. It is a choice to go down a path of emptiness, frustration, and misery, ultimately towards self-destruction. It is a path of belligerent denial and pathological dishonesty where we fail to treat the disease because it's easier to cling to the comforting lie that nothing's wrong.

The false story is the one that says we are advancing and evolving in a positive way. Media screen-feeds us the feel-good lie that we progress and advance and get better with each new generation. Screens all around us reinforce the lie during nearly every waking moment. We *have no choice* but to believe it. The lie feels good. Because of screen-suggestibility, "feels good" equals "true." The absurd advance-as-a-species story, however, is the most dangerous lie, and the most fraudulent mythology.

Hope for the Future and a Brighter Tomorrow

While the outlook for society appears dark and not likely to brighten in the near future, there is still a lot of hope for individuals. Anyone can decide to be an exception to the rule. Replacing passive screentime with active participation in life gets easier after a little progress. *The Motivation Myth* author Jeff Haden's insight is not oversimplified, it is just profoundly simple: "A productive body in motion tends to stay in productive motion."[285]

There are tactics to help switch from passive stagnation to active achievement gradually. Focusing on one small change at a time, repeating active habits with tiny increases over time, attaching a new good habit to an existing routine ("stacking habits"), are ways to get started (from *Exist* co-founder Belle Beth Cooper's story).[286]

One of our most important choices in life will be whether to settle for the "as is" self of being "only human," or rise to the "can be" self to become "fully human." Change gradually, or change all at once, but change!

Hope comes from desire: Push the pain threshold towards fulfillment. Success comes from taking the high road of strength and action. Put away the screen and carry the torch.

PART III: Postscript

AUTHOR'S NOTES

My first exposure to studies on TV's damage came from reading Dr. Winn's *Plug-In Drug* in 1981. But long before I read *Plug-In Drug*, I had already stopped watching TV. I picked up Winn's book out of curiosity to see if my impression of TV matched up with her book.

It did. My impression of TV was confirmed by scientific study almost forty years ago, and by countless more studies since then. My perception of TV's harmfulness and my normal common sense were all I needed. That's all anyone should need.

Unfortunately, common sense is one of the casualties of a passive screen-centric lifestyle. After a moment's reflection, however, I think we all have the same inkling of the screen's unhealthy effects. Haven't we admitted it every time we've said "I watch too much TV"?[287]

Very often we watch a lot of TV, but say "I really don't watch that much TV." We really believe it, because TV is such a thief of time. We watch TV for five hours, and the next day we swear that we only "watched about an hour of TV last night." The other two or three hours of free time were spent on social media and other screens, mostly consuming video on several devices. Screentime is virtually unconscious time, except we are soaking in countless messages that quietly shape our brain during that evaporated time. Hence the screenformation of our minds and our culture.

Anxiety about Death: Where Did the Time Go?

In the past, by age 75, people were weary with life, with no anxiety about dying of old age. They lived long enough and they felt it inside. Today's people are different. By age 75 we will suffer terrible anxiety at the thought of dying, because to us it seems like we only lived 25 years. "How can life be over so soon?!" In a way, that impression is correct. TV-viewers really lived only 25 of their 75 years. At age 75 we will have the life experience that a 25-year-old had in the past. We spent 50 of those years watching screens and failing to develop.

In the past, if we asked 300 million people what they did with their lives, we got 300 million different answers. Today when we ask 300 million people what they did with their lives, we get one answer: "I watched everything on a screen."

Where Are the Greats?

Where are all the greats like those we hear about from the past? Where are today's versions of yesterday's Faulkners and Hemmingways and Angelous, the Benjamin Franklins and Mark Twains, the Albert Einsteins and Thomas Edisons, the Vincent van Goghs and Leonardo da Vincis, the George Washingtons and Abraham Lincolns, the Martin Luthers and Martin Luther Kings, the Mozarts and Bachs, the Louis Armstrongs and Benny Goodmans, the Louis Pasteurs and Jane Goodalls, the Andrés Segovias and Isaac Sterns, the Ginger Rogers and Fred Astaires, the Buffalo Bills and Annie Oakleys, the Orson Welles and Alfred Hitchcocks, the Arthur Conan Doyles and Agatha Christies, the Eddie Rickenbackers and Amelia Earharts, the Henry Fords and Walt Disneys?

The answer is: They grew up passively entertained by screen devices, mindlessly consuming video, playing screen games, with mindless time-drains like social media, instead of becoming great.

The potential greats of today had special potential, but they did not become special.

Potentially great people have relinquished greatness in favor of passive screen entertainment. It didn't happen by choice, it happened because of being born into a culture that is immersed in screens. There was no choice. Day by day, hour by hour, screentime systematically drained the strength and hope out of those who might've become great in the past forty or fifty years. Upon a once-adventure-filled road of life, the roadside is littered with deflated skills, dead potentials, unfinished accomplishments, dreams up in smoke, culture in ashes.

Even early TV stars note that they honed their craft because they had to entertain themselves in their own pre-screen days. For example, TV icon Dick Van Dyke recalls, "We got together and harmonized, told jokes, and invented tall tales that kept us amused. We spent hours exercising our imaginations and entertaining ourselves in those days before television and long before the Internet."[288] TV stars with pre-screen childhoods look around them, and don't like what they see in their own profession. *Columbo* star Peter Falk, for example, talked about, "my contempt for much of what is seen on TV—my refusal to deal with mindless action, dumb jokes, and exposition posing as real talk."[289]

As the years go by, we have to keep looking farther and farther back to find anything developed and well done, let alone heroic or brilliant. Everything is reduced to mediocrity. Lions of public service and the arts are relegated to history books and museums. They have an alien feel about them, unfamiliar and difficult to imagine. This endangered species will soon become extinct without much notice.

Final Thought

For parents especially, consider the tragedy of wiping out all of your child's real-world and rewarding experiences and life skills, and replacing them with incompetence and shallow screen-memories.

Step back and look at it objectively. You are equipped with the knowledge of the scientific proof about the effects of screentime on child development. You are up above the rooftops looking down into the average American household. You see two 30-year-old parents and their 3-year-old child. Each day of the year, those parents must make a choice:

A. Nurture the child's mental functioning, mental health, emotional development, and physical health; or

B. Damage the child's mental functioning, mental health, emotional development, and physical health.

Now ask the question about those two 30-year-old parents: Each year, how many of the 365 days do you think the parents should choose A? How many of the 365 days do you think the parents should choose B?

Now step back into your own life. Your child's potential is in your hands: A or B? Every day. The choice is that simple.

AUTHOR BIOGRAPHY

Robert Rose-Coutré has been studying people and taking notes since earliest memory. Starting at a young age, he spent his life studying people, society, history, and other cultures. Since early childhood he sought out older people to learn as much as possible about older generations. Some of his earliest boyhood memories included talking with World War I veterans or anyone born in the 1800s to learn what life was like in the old days. Those experiences brought home how precious people are, that the old-school ways of fully-human living should not be dismissed and lost so easily. His motivation has been to learn about human feeling, thinking, and behavior; understanding relationships, appreciating people, and leading a meaningful life that benefits others.

Robert Rose-Coutré has a Master of Arts degree in literature, with additional graduate studies in philosophy. He studied analytical philosophy, language, and logic. Rose-Coutré has been a member of high-IQ societies such as American Mensa, ISI-Society, World Intelligence Network, Intertel, and Ronald K. Hoeflin Societies.

Careerwise, Rose-Coutré has been a digital marketer, editor, writer, and publisher. He previously published a book of commentary on active living; a scholarly book on works of art, abstract objects, and the philosophy of language; and a novel exploring the fragmented condition of marriage and the effects of emptiness in modern society.

Robert Rose-Coutré is grateful to have had a TV growing up, having watched enough to gain an intimate understand its effects, but limited enough not to do too much damage. He is grateful to his parents for those strict limits. Because of that limitation, he had time for a lot of activities that leave him with precious memories of old-style living.

With that extra 20,000-plus hours of childhood and teenage development, he grew up reading novels, reading every volume of his family's encyclopedias along with many other books on science and history; played long hours of football, baseball, basketball, soccer, tennis, and golf; sold newspapers at a shopping center at age 9 and had many jobs growing up; did yardwork and household chores most every day, always on Saturday; learned household maintenance like replacing fixtures, roofing, dry walling, painting houses inside and out, welding, metalworking, woodworking; rode a bicycle everywhere many miles a day including to and from school and jobs (parents didn't give rides); became a competitive speed skater at the local roller-skating rink at age 10; got in fights with kids in the neighborhood; started a daily exercise regimen at age 13 (and kept it up ever since); learned how to play the organ from his grandmother; took guitar lessons; won or placed in small local tournaments in chess, billiards, and ping-pong, and played those games regularly; learned sailing, motorboating, rowing, canoeing, and water-skiing; learned martial arts, juggling, knife-throwing, target shooting, archery, and horseback riding; learned endurance swimming and lifesaving and became a lifeguard at age 16; camped on weekends once a month and learned skills in camping, wilderness survival, and many other outdoors skills; worked through the ranks of scouting and earned Eagle Scout; participated in community service projects through scouting and church; and enjoyed almost all recreation time with friends, doing things in the real world with real people, growing and learning how to be a human, an old-school human, fully human.

Today, we trade all that for passive screen shallowness and a dull lifetime of effortless emptiness.

LINKS TO COMPANION PAGES

- Website:
  http://www.screenformation.com

- Facebook:
  https://www.facebook.com/Screenformation

- Twitter:
  https://twitter.com/screenformation

Key to the Term "Screenformation"

The term "Screenformation" has two complementary meanings:

1. The literal meaning from Screen and Formation: The changed formation of the mind itself, resulting from screentime. Instead of natural mind formation, minds adopt Screenformation (reduced brain activity and altered perception of reality).

2. The portmanteau of Screen and Information, or Screen-Information. This is information received into the mind from screens. Instead of information, minds receive only Screenformation (a shallow facsimile of information, or "information lite"). The shallow medium fools us into thinking we have become informed.

PART IV:
Works Consulted and End Notes

WORKS CONSULTED

Achor, Shawn. "The Happy Secret to Better Work" *Ted Talk*. February, 2012. https://www.ted.com/talks/shawn_achor_the_happy_secret_to_better_work/transcript?language=en.

Alter, Adam. "Tech Bigwigs Know How Addictive Their Products Are. Why Don't the Rest of Us?" *Wired.com*. https://www.wired.com/2017/03/irresistible-the-rise-of-addictive-technology-and-the-business-of-keeping-us-hooked/, March 24, 2017.

Anderson, Porter. "Study: Multitasking is counterproductive" *CNN*. http://www.cnn.com/2001/CAREER/trends/08/05/multitasking.study/index.html

Angelou, Maya, quoted in *Maya Angelou: 365 Quotes and Sayings of Phenomenal Woman*, by Maura Craig. (quote #348). Sep 27, 2014. Google digitized version: https://books.google.com/books?id=UKiiBAAAQBAJ&pg=PT73.

Aristotle. *BrainyQuote.com*, Xplore Inc, 2014. http://www.brainyquote.com/quotes/quotes/a/aristotle132211.html, accessed September 16, 2014.

Aristotle. *Goodreads*. http://www.goodreads.com/quotes/31240-happiness-is-a-state-of-activity, July 24, 2015.

Arum, Richard. "College Graduates: Satisfied, but Adrift" in *The State of the American Mind*. p. 73, Mark Bauerlein and Adam Bellow, eds. West Conshohocken, PA: Templeton, 2015.

Becker-Phelps, Leslie. "Don't Just React: Choose Your Response" *Psychology Today*. https://www.psychologytoday.com/blog/making-change/201307/dont-just-react-choose-your-response, July 23, 2013.

Berger, Eric. "By 2010 most science Ph.D.s will go to foreign-born students" *SciGuy*. http://blog.chron.com/sciguy/2007/11/by-2010-most-science-ph-d-s-will-go-to-foreign-born-students/, November 21, 2007

Bernstein, Emily E. and Richard J. McNally. "Acute aerobic exercise helps overcome emotion regulation deficits" *Cognition and Emotion*, DOI: 10.1080/02699931.2016.1168284 http://dx.doi.org/10.1080/02699931.2016.1168284, April 4, 2016.

Birdsong, Kristina. "This is Your Child's Brain on TV" *Scientific Learning*. http://www.scilearn.com/blog/how-television-impacts-learning, Mar 22, 2016.

Blachowicz, James. "There Is No Scientific Method" *The Stone, New York Times*. http://www.nytimes.com/2016/07/04/opinion/there-is-no-scientific-method.html, July 4, 2016.

Boyse, Kyla. "Television and Children" *Michigan Medicine* (University of Michigan). http://www.med.umich.edu/yourchild/topics/tv.htm, August 2010.

Bradberry, Travis and Jean Greaves. *Emotional Intelligence 2.0* (San Diego, California: TalentSmart, 2009).
- Bradberry, Travis. "9 Habits of Profoundly Influential People". https://www.linkedin.com/pulse/critical-habits-profoundly-influential-people-dr-travis-bradberry/, July 20, 2015.
- Bradberry, Travis. "9 Surprising Things Ultra Productive People Do Every Day". https://www.linkedin.com/pulse/surprising-things-ultra-productive-people-do-every-day-bradberry/, November 7, 2016.
- Bradberry, Travis. "11 Things Ultra-Productive People Do Differently" *Forbes*. https://www.forbes.com/sites/travisbradberry/2015/05/13/11-things-ultra-productive-people-do-differently/, May 13, 2015.
- Bradberry, Travis. "12 Habits of Genuine People". https://www.linkedin.com/pulse/importance-being-genuine-dr-travis-bradberry/, November 15, 2015.

- Bradberry, Travis. "13 Habits of Exceptionally Likeable People". https://www.linkedin.com/pulse/13-habits-exceptionally-likeable-people-dr-travis-bradberry, January 27, 2015.
- Bradberry, Travis. "13 Things Mentally Strong People Won't Do". https://www.linkedin.com/pulse/13-things-mentally-strong-people-wont-do-dr-travis-bradberry/, September 11, 2017.
- Bradberry, Travis. "Eight Habits of Considerate People". https://www.linkedin.com/pulse/eight-habits-considerate-people-dr-travis-bradberry, November 8, 2017.
- Bradberry, Travis. "These are the habits that mentally strong people rely on" *World Economic Forum.* https://www.weforum.org/agenda/2016/10/habits-to-help-you-develop-mental-strength, October 26, 2016.

Bryson, Carey. "Babies and TV: Is Screen Time Good for Your Little One?" *ThoughtCo.* https://www.thoughtco.com/should-babies-watch-tv-2107982, June 22, 2017.

Buckner, Candace. "NBA players know they're addicted to their phones. Good luck getting them to unplug" *The Washington Post.* https://www.washingtonpost.com/sports/nba-players-know-theyre-addicted-to-their-phones-good-luck-getting-them-to-unplug/2018/03/19/6165cb96-2563-11e8-b79d-f3d931db7f68_story.html, March 19, 2018.

"Carbon footprint" *Wikipedia.* http://en.wikipedia.org/wiki/Carbon_footprint, accessed November 1, 2014.

Carey, Kevin. "Americans Think We Have the World's Best Colleges. We Don't." *The New York Times.* https://www.nytimes.com/2014/06/29/upshot/americans-think-we-have-the-worlds-best-colleges-we-dont.html, June 28, 2014.

"Children who watch 'excessive' amounts of TV are more likely to have criminal convictions, exhibit aggression and experience negative emotions: study." *New York Daily News*. http://www.nydailynews.com/life-style/health/kids-watch-excessive-tv-criminal-convictions-young-adulthood-study-article-1.1267868, February 19, 2013.

Christensen, Allan Stromfeldt. "Lemminged: to be herded off the peak oil cliff by filmmakers" *TransitionVoice.com*. http://transitionvoice.com/2014/11/lemminged-to-be-herded-off-the-peak-oil-cliff-by-filmmakers/, November 11, 2014.

Chua, Celestine. "Top 10 Reasons You Should Stop Watching TV" *Personal Excellence: Be Your Best Self, Live Your Best Life.* http://personalexcellence.co/blog/top-10-reasons-you-should-stop-watching-tv/, May 2, 2010

Cicero, Marcus Tullius. *De Oratore,* Book II §36. The Loeb Classical Library, English translation Cambridge, Massachusetts, Harvard University Press, 1967. https://archive.org/stream/cicerodeoratore01ciceuoft/cicerodeoratore01ciceuoft_djvu.txt, 55 BC.

Constine, Josh. "Jeff Bezos' guide to life" *TechCrunch.* https://techcrunch.com/2017/11/05/jeff-bezos-guide-to-life/, November 5, 2017.

Cooper, Belle Beth. "How to Be a Success at Everything" *Fast Company*. https://www.fastcompany.com/3056613/how-i-became-a-morning-person-read-more-books-and-learned-, February 12, 2016.

Courogen, Carrie. "9 Harsh Realities About Graduating College That I Wish Someone Had Warned Me About" *Bustle*. https://www.bustle.com/articles/80461-9-harsh-realities-about-graduating-college-that-i-wish-someone-had-warned-me-about, May 4, 2015.

Dahl, Melissa. "How Neuroscientists Explain the Mind-Clearing Magic of Running" Science of Us, *New York Magazine*. http://nymag.com/scienceofus/2016/04/how-neuroscientists-explain-the-mind-clearing-magic-of-running.html, April 21, 2016.

Disraeli, Benjamin, Earl of Beaconsfield, quoted in *Puck*, Volume XV, No. 370 (p. 95). April 9, 1884. Google digitized version: https://books.google.com/books?id=0_kiAQAAMAAJ&pg=PA95.

Doverspike, William F., Ph.D. "How To Make Yourself Miserable: Discovering the Secrets to Unhappiness" *Georgia Psychological Association*. Atlanta. http://gapsychology.org/displaycommon.cfm?an=1&subarticlenbr=341, accessed September 29, 2014.

Dovey, Ceridwen. "Can Reading Make You Happier?" *The New Yorker*. http://www.newyorker.com/culture/cultural-comment/can-reading-make-you-happier, June 9, 2015.

Dunning, David. "We Are All Confident Idiots" *Pacific Standard*. https://www3.nd.edu/~ghaeffel/ConfidentIdiots.pdf, October 27, 2014.

Dunning, David and Justin Kruger. "Unskilled and Unaware of It: How Difficulties in Recognizing One's Own Incompetence Lead to Inflated Self-Assessments" *Journal of Personality and Social Psychology.* 1999, Vol. 77, No. 6, 1121-1134. Cornell University. http://psych.colorado.edu/~vanboven/teaching/p7536_heurbias/p7536_readings/kruger_dunning.pdf

Ecclesiastes Chapter 7, verses 4 and 5. *The New Oxford Annotated Bible* (New York: Oxford University Press, 1977, Revised Standard Version) p. 810.

Educational Testing Service (ETS). "America's Skills Challenge: Millennials and the Future" *The ETS Center for Research on Human Capital and Education.* Princeton, NJ: January 2015. https://www.ets.org/s/research/30079/asc-millennials-and-the-future.pdf.

Falk, Peter. *Just One More Thing*. (New York: Carroll & Graf, 2007) pp. 165–166.

Fields, Douglas. "Watching TV Alters Children's Brain Structure and Lowers IQ". http://rdouglasfields.com/2015/05/watching-tv-alters-childrens-brain-structure-and-lowers-iq/, May 4, 2015.

Fisher, Matthew et al. "Searching for Explanations: How the Internet Inflates Estimates of Internal Knowledge" *Journal of Experimental Psychology* 144(3). pp. 674–687, June 2015.

Fox, EJ and Mike Spies. "Who Was America's Most Well-Spoken President?" *Vocativ*. http://www.vocativ.com/interactive/usa/us-politics/presidential-readability/, October 10, 2014.

"Fred Astaire Dancer (1899–1987)" *The Biography.com website*. https://www.biography.com/people/fred-astaire-9190991, Last Updated, April 27, 2017.

Frey, Bruno S.; Christine Benesch; Alois Stutzer. "Does watching TV make us happy?" *Journal of Economic Psychology* Volume 28, Issue 3, June 2007. Elsevier B.V. (ScienceDirect.com). http://www.bsfrey.ch/articles/459_07.pdf, February 14, 2007.

Frierson, William. "Dream vs. Reality: What Happens After Graduation" *College Recruiter*. https://www.collegerecruiter.com/blog/2015/07/14/dream-vs-reality-what-happens-after-graduation/, July 14, 2015.

Gardner, Amanda. "TV watching raises risk of health problems, dying young" *CNN*. http://www.cnn.com/2011/HEALTH/06/14/tv.watching.unhealthy/, June 14, 2011.

"Gender Switch: When Did Men Become So Feminine?" *Urban Belle*. http://urbanbellemag.com/2010/10/gender-switch-when-did-men-become-so-feminine.html, October 18, 2010

Goldsmith, Belinda. "Watching hours of TV daily could shorten your life – study" Ed. Miral Fahmy. *Reuters*. http://in.reuters.com/article/worldNews/idINIndia-45316820100111, January 12, 2010.

Gollwitzer, Peter M., et al., "When Intentions Go Public: Does Social Reality Widen the Intention-Behavior Gap?" *Psychological Science* 20, no. 5 (May 1, 2009): 612. http://journals.sagepub.com/doi/abs/10.1111/j.1467-9280.2009.02336.x, May 1, 2009.

Grabmeier, Jeff. "Both liberals, conservatives can have science bias: Study finds different topics bedevil the left and right" *The Ohio State University*. https://news.osu.edu/news/2015/02/09/both-liberals-conservatives-can-have-science-bias/, February 09, 2015.

Ha, Thu-Huong. "New research links reading books with longer life" *Quartz*. http://qz.com/754109/new-research-links-reading-books-with-longer-life/, August 10, 2016.

Haden, Jeff. *The Motivation Myth.* New York: Penguin, 2018.

Hamilton, Jon. "How Play Wires Kids' Brains For Social and Academic Success" *KQED News.* KQED.org, National Public Radio (NPR), Copyright 2014. http://ww2.kqed.org/mindshift/2014/08/07/how-play-wires-kids-brains-for-social-and-academic-success/, August 7, 2014.

Healy, Jane M. "Endangered Minds" *Creating the Future: Perspectives on Educational Change*. Ed. Dee Dickinson. Johns Hopkins University. 2012. http://education.jhu.edu/PD/newhorizons/future/creating_the_future/cr fut_healy.cfm.

Healy, Jane M. *Endangered Minds: Why Children Don't Think And What We Can Do About It*. Simon & Schuster, 1999.

Heilbrunn Timeline of Art History. The Metropolitan Museum of Art. http://www.metmuseum.org/toah/hd/gogh/hd_gogh.htm, July, 30 2015.

Henderson, Emma. "Watching lots of TV 'makes you stupid'" *The Independent*.
http://www.independent.co.uk/news/science/watching-lots-of-tv-makes-you-stupid-says-american-universities-a6759026.html, December 3, 2015.

Heshmat, Shahram. "What Is Confirmation Bias?" *Psychology Today*.
https://www.psychologytoday.com/blog/science-choice/201504/what-is-confirmation-bias, April 23, 2015.

Hickman, Martin. "Watching TV 'makes toddlers less intelligent'" *The Independent*.
http://www.independent.co.uk/news/education/education-news/watching-tv-makes-toddlers-less-intelligent-1960856.html, May 2, 2010.

Higgins, E. Tory. "Self-Discrepancy Theory" *Advances in Experimental Social Psychology*, Volume 22. Leonard Berkowitz, ed. (Cambridge, Massachusetts: Academic Press. March 28, 1989) pp. 93–135 (specific referenced quotes on pp. 118–119).

Hill, David L. "Why to Avoid TV Before Age 2" (early brain development). *American Academy of Pediatrics*.
http://www.healthychildren.org/English/family-life/Media/Pages/Why-to-Avoid-TV-Before-Age-2.aspx, May 11, 2013.
Original Source: Dad to Dad: Parenting Like a Pro (Copyright © American Academy of Pediatrics 2012).

Hinckley, David. "Average American watches 5 hours of TV per day, report shows Time spent watching live TV increases steadily as we get older, according to a new report from Nielsen" *New York Daily News*.
http://nydn.us/1fHRJee, March 5, 2014.

Hoang, Tina D., MSPH; Jared Reis, PhD; Na Zhu, MD, MPH; David R. Jacobs Jr, PhD; Lenore J. Launer, PhD; Rachel A. Whitmer, PhD; Stephen Sidney, MD; Kristine Yaffe, MD. "Effect of Early Adult Patterns of Physical Activity and Television Viewing on Midlife Cognitive Function" *JAMA Psychiatry* (The Journal of the American Medical Association).
http://archpsyc.jamanetwork.com/article.aspx?articleid=2471270, January 2016, Vol 73, No. 1.

Holthaus, Eric and Chris Kirk. "A Filthy History: Interactive map: Which countries have emitted the most carbon since 1850?" *Slate.com*. http://www.slate.com/articles/technology/future_tense/2014/05/carbon _dioxide_emissions_by_country_over_time_the_worst_global_warming_ polluters.html.

"HOME-SCHOOLING: Outstanding results on national tests" *The Washington Times*. http://www.washingtontimes.com/news/2009/aug/30/home-schooling-outstanding-results-national-tests/, August 30, 2009.

"How Satellites Work With Mobile Phones" *CompareMyMobile*. http://blog.comparemymobile.com/how-satellites-work-with-mobile-phones/, accessed December 21, 2017.

Hu, Elise. "Facebook Makes Us Sadder And Less Satisfied, Study Finds" *National Public Radio*. http://www.npr.org/blogs/alltechconsidered/2013/08/19/213568763/res earchers-facebook-makes-us-sadder-and-less-satisfied, August 20, 2013.

Hyodo, Kazuki and Ippeita Dan, Yasushi Kyutoku, Kazuya Suwabe, Kyeongho Byun, Genta Ochi, Morimasa Kato, Hideaki Soya. "The association between aerobic fitness and cognitive function in older men mediated by frontal lateralization" *NeuroImage*, v. 125, pp. 291–300, January 15, 2016.

"I'm Addicted to Television": The Personality, Imagination, and TV Watching Patterns of Self-Identified TV Addicts. Robert D. McIlwraith in *Journal of Broadcasting and Electronic Media*, Vol. 42, No. 3, pages 371-- 386; Summer 1998.

Ingraham, Christopher. "Today's men are not nearly as strong as their dads were, researchers say" *Washington Post*. https://www.washingtonpost.com/news/wonk/wp/2016/08/15/todays-men-are-nowhere-near-as-strong-as-their-dads-were-researchers-say/, August 15, 2016.

Jacobs, Tom. "Searching the Internet Creates an Illusion of Knowledge" *Pacific Standard online.* https://psmag.com/environment/searching-internet-creates-the-illusion-of-knowledge-, April 1, 2015.

Jaschik, Scott. "Let the Right Ones In" *Slate.com.* http://www.slate.com/articles/life/inside_higher_ed/2014/10/college_ad missions_rose_hulman_institute_of_technology_uses_locus_of_control.h tml, October 30, 2014.

Jayson, Sharon. "Generation Y's goal? Wealth and fame" *USA Today.* http://usatoday30.usatoday.com/news/nation/2007-01-09-gen-y-cover_x.htm, Posted January 9,2007, Updated January 10, 2007.

Jordan, Alexander H., Benoît Monin, Carol S. Dweck, Benjamin J. Lovett, Oliver P. John, and James J. Gross. "Misery Has More Company Than People Think: Underestimating the Prevalence of Others' Negative Emotions". *Personality and Social Psychology Bulletin* January 2011 37: 120-135. National Institutes of Health. http://www.ncbi.nlm.nih.gov/pmc/articles/PMC4138214/, January 2011, latest update August 19, 2014.

Joyce, Amy. "How helicopter parents are ruining college students" *The Washington Post.* http://www.washingtonpost.com/news/parenting/wp/2014/09/02/how-helicopter-parents-are-ruining-college-students/, September 2, 2014

Kennedy-Moore, Eileen. "Do Boys Need Rough and Tumble Play?" *Psychology Today.* https://www.psychologytoday.com/blog/growing-friendships/201506/do-boys-need-rough-and-tumble-play, June 30, 2015.

Keohane, Joe. "How Facts Backfire: Researchers Discover a Surprising Threat to Democracy: Our Brains" *Boston Globe online.* http://archive.boston.com/bostonglobe/ideas/articles/2010/07/11/how_facts_backfire/, July 11, 2010.

Knott, Stephen, ed. "Life Before the Presidency" *American President: George Washington (1732–1799), Essays on George Washington and His Administration*. Miller Center, University of Virginia. http://millercenter.org/president/washington/essays/biography/2, accessed November 19, 2014.

Krieger, Richard Alan. *Civilization's Quotations: Life's Ideal.* (New York: Algora Publishing, 2002) p. 122.

Kross, Ethan; Philippe Verduyn, Emre Demiralp, Jiyoung Park, David Seungjae Lee, Natalie Lin, Holly Shablack, John Jonides, Oscar Ybarra. "Facebook Use Predicts Declines in Subjective Well-Being in Young Adults" *PLoS ONE* 8(8): e69841. doi:10.1371/journal.pone.0069841. http://www.plosone.org/article/info%3Adoi%2F10.1371%2Fjournal.pone.0069841, August 14, 2013.

Krugman, Herbert E. "Brain Wave Measures of Media Involvement" *How Advertising Works: The Role of Research.* (New York SAGE Publications, 1998) pp. 139–151.

Krugman, Herbert E., and Eugene L. Hartley. "Passive Learning From Television" *The Public Opinion Quarterly,* Vol. 34, No. 2. (Oxford University Press, 1970) pp. 184-190.

Kubey, Robert and Mihaly Csikszentmihalyi. "Television Addiction is no mere metaphor" *Scientific American*. http://www.academia.edu/5065840/Television_Addiction_is_no_mere_metaphor, accessed January 23, 2016.

Kubey, Robert and Mihaly Csikszentmihalyi. *Television and the Quality of Life: How Viewing Shapes Everyday Experience.* Lawrence Erlbaum Associates, 1990.

Kubey, Robert; Michael J. Lavin and John R. Barrows. "Internet Use and Collegiate Academic Performance Decrements: Early Findings". *Journal of Communication*, Vol. 51, No. 2, pages 366--382; June 2001.

Lang, Annie. The Limited Capacity Model of Mediated Message Processing. *Journal of Communication*, Vol. 50, No. 1, pages 46--70; March 2000.

Leonard, Tom. "'Passive' TV Can Harm Your Baby's Speech Making It Harder for Them to Later Cope In School" *Daily Mail*. http://www.dailymail.co.uk/news/article-2054950/Passive-TV-watching-harm-babies-speech.html, October 28, 2011.

MacBeth, Tannis M., ed. Television Dependence, Diagnosis, and Prevention. Robert W. Kubey in Tuning in to Young Viewers: Social Science Perspectives on Television. Sage, 1995.

McCarthy, Caroline. "Hulu: We're evil, and proud of it" *CNet*. https://www.cnet.com/news/hulu-were-evil-and-proud-of-it/, February 2, 2009.

Michel, Dan, *Remorse of Conscience*, or *Ayenbite of inwyt*, ed. Richard Morris (London: N. Trubner & Co., 1895) pp. 74-75. Morris' 1895 republication is from Michel's 1340 translation from French to Kentish. Michel's 1340 translation is of the 13th century French *Somme le Roi*. My quote is from a translation of the 1340 Kentish into modern English, translation by Judith G. Humphries, in "The Personification of Death in Middle English Literature" (Denton, Texas: 1970, North Texas State University) p. 10.

"Masculine And Feminine Roles In Relationships Sociology Essay" *Essays, UK*. http://www.ukessays.com/essays/sociology/masculine-and-feminine-roles-in-relationships-sociology-essay.php?cref=1, November 2013.

Mooney, Chris. "Liberals deny science, too" *The Washington Post*. https://www.washingtonpost.com/news/wonk/wp/2014/10/28/liberals-deny-science-too/, October 28, 2014.

Morrow, Jon. "How to Be Smart in a World of Dumb Bloggers" *BoostBlogTraffic*. http://boostblogtraffic.com/smart-blogger/, September 17, 2013.

Morrow, Jon. "On Gluttony, Selfishness, and Unleashing the Power Within" *BoostBlogTraffic*. http://boostblogtraffic.com/unleash-your-power/, November 27, 2014.

Newman, Virginia. *Digging into Food Waste.* "Students from the Wenatchee School District take a closer look at the food served in their cafeteria, from the farm to the kitchen to the trays to the trash cans." https://youtu.be/91vU6DLHMPs, Published October 20, 2015.

Nichols, Tom. *The Death of Expertise.* New York: Oxford University Press, 2017.

Nielsen. "Percentage of Americans who say they watch too much TV: 49 %" *BLS American Time Use Survey*, A.C. Nielsen Co. http://www.statisticbrain.com/television-watching-statistics/, Date Verified: 12.7.2013 (July 12, 2013).

Nielsen. "Television, Internet and Mobile Usage in the U.S. — A2/M2 Three Screen Report 4th Quarter 2008". Copyright © 2009 The Nielsen Company. http://i.cdn.turner.com/cnn/2009/images/02/24/screen.press.b.pdf, accessed May 29, 2014.

Panksepp, Jaak. "Can PLAY diminish ADHD and facilitate the construction of the social brain?" *Journal of the Canadian Academy of Child and Adolescent Psychiatry* (16, 57-66), 2007.

Park, Alice. "Baby Einsteins: Not So Smart After All" *Time.* http://content.time.com/time/health/article/0,8599,1650352,00.html, August 06, 2007.

Pellis, Sergio M., and Vivien C. Pellis. "Rough-and-Tumble Play: Training and Using the Social Brain" *The Oxford Handbook of the Development of Play* (December 2010).
Online Reference:
http://www.oxfordhandbooks.com/view/10.1093/oxfordhb/9780195393002.001.0001/oxfordhb-9780195393002-e-019, September 2012.

"Physical Fighting by Youth" *Child Trends Databank.* https://www.childtrends.org/indicators/physical-fighting-by-youth/, Accessed December 23, 2017.

Pickersgill, Eric. *Removed.* http://www.removed.social/, accessed October 21, 2015.

"Planet or Plastic? A Brief History of How Plastic Has Changed Our World" *National Geographic.* https://video.nationalgeographic.com/video/magazine/planet-or-plastic/180516-ngm-brief-history-of-plastic, Accessed May 18, 2018.

Quast, Lisa. "Why Grit Is More Important Than IQ When You're Trying To Become Successful" *Forbes.* https://www.forbes.com/sites/lisaquast/2017/03/06/why-grit-is-more-important-than-iq-when-youre-trying-to-become-successful/, March 6, 2017.

Rampell, Catherine. "The rise of the 'gentleman's A' and the GPA arms race" *The Washington Post.* https://www.washingtonpost.com/opinions/the-rise-of-the-gentlemans-a-and-the-gpa-arms-race/2016/03/28/05c9e966-f522-11e5-9804-537defcc3cf6_story.html, March 28, 2016.

Redden, Elizabeth. "Foreign Student Dependence" *Inside Higher Education.* https://www.insidehighered.com/news/2013/07/12/new-report-shows-dependence-us-graduate-programs-foreign-students, July 12, 2013.

Richtel, Matt. "The Myth of Multitasking" *Attached to Technology and Paying a Price*, p. 2. http://www.nytimes.com/2010/06/07/technology/07brain.html, June 6, 2010.

Roosevelt, Franklin Delano. *AZQuotes.* http://www.azquotes.com/quote/250883.

Rothman, Johanna. "Why Multitasking Doesn't Work" *Pragmatic Manager.* http://www.jrothman.com/2011/01/why-multitasking-doesnt-work/, January 1, 2011.

Ryan, Claudine. "Why is watching TV so bad for you?" *ABC Health & Wellbeing.* http://www.abc.net.au/health/thepulse/stories/2014/07/24/4043618.htm, July 24, 2014.

Schulte, Brigid. *Overwhelmed: Work, Love, and Play When No One Has the Time.* New York: Simon & Schuster, Inc./Sarah Crichton Books, 2014.

Schuman, Rebecca. "Welcome to 13th Grade!" *Slate.com.* http://www.slate.com/articles/life/education/2014/10/high_schools_offe r_a_fifth_year_of_high_school_13th_grade_is_a_great_idea.html October 22, 2014.

Schwartz, Mel. "Is Our Society Manufacturing Depressed People?" *Psychology Today.* https://www.psychologytoday.com/blog/shift-mind/201203/is-our-society-manufacturing-depressed-people, March 19, 2012.

Sigman, Aric. "How TV Is (Quite Literally) Killing Us" *Daily Mail.* http://www.whale.to/b/sigman.html, Oct 1, 2005.

Smith, Peter K. "Chapter 6: Physical Activity Play: Exercise Play and Rough-and-Tumble" *Children and Play* (April 2009). Online Reference: http://onlinelibrary.wiley.com/doi/10.1002/9781444311006.ch6/summar y, April 24, 2009.

Sornson, Bob. "Who's Looking Out for the Children?" *Early Learning Foundation.* http://earlylearningfoundation.com/whos-looking-out-for-the-children/, accessed March 18, 2017.

Stillman, Jessica. "Complaining Is Terrible for You, According to Science" *Inc.com.* http://www.inc.com/jessica-stillman/complaining-rewires-your-brain-for-negativity-science-says.html, February 29, 2016.

Stillman, Jessica. "The Cold, Hard Truth: You're Overwhelmed Because You Want to Be" *Inc.com.* http://www.inc.com/jessica-stillman/cure-for-feeling-overwhelmed-is-to-stop-talking-about-it.html, March 28, 2014.

Stillman, Jessica. "Which Country Has the Most Productive Workers?" *Inc.com.*
http://www.inc.com/jessica-stillman/which-country-has-the-most-productive-workers.html, July 25, 2014.

Strasburger, Victor C., MD, FAAP, and Marjorie J. Hogan, MD, FAAP. "Children, Adolescents, and the Media". American Academy of Pediatrics. http://pediatrics.aappublications.org/content/132/5/958.full, May 11, 2013.

Stromberg, Joseph. "Why you should take notes by hand — not on a laptop". *Vox: Science & Health.*
http://www.vox.com/2014/6/4/5776804/note-taking-by-hand-versus-laptop, March 31, 2015.

Szalavitz, Maia. "Misery Has More Company Than You Think, Especially on Facebook". *Time.*
http://healthland.time.com/2011/01/27/youre-not-alone-misery-has-more-company-than-you-think/, January 27, 2011.

Takeuchi, Hikaru; Yasuyuki Taki; Hiroshi Hashizume; Kohei Asano; Michiko Asano; Yuko Sassa; Susumu Yokota; Yuka Kotozaki; Rui Nouchi; and Ryuta Kawashima. "The Impact of Television Viewing on Brain Structures: Cross-Sectional and Longitudinal Analyses" *Cerebral Cortex,* Oxford Journals. https://cercor.oxfordjournals.org/content/early/2013/11/18/cercor.bht3 15.full, April 15, 2015.

Taylor, Jim. "Parenting: The Sad Misuse of Self-esteem" *Psychology Today.* https://www.psychologytoday.com/blog/the-power-prime/201002/parenting-the-sad-misuse-self-esteem, February 22, 2010.

Taylor, Jim. "Pro Athletes are Hooked on Social Media Too" http://www.drjimtaylor.com/4.0/pro-athletes-are-hooked-on-social-media-too/, accessed April 23, 2018.

"Television Addiction" *All About Life Challenges.*
http://www.allaboutlifechallenges.org/television-addiction.htm, accessed September 21, 2014.

"Television History - The First 75 Years" *TVhistory.TV.* © 2001-2013. http://www.tvhistory.tv/facts-stats.htm.

"Television: Opiate of the Masses". *FamilyResource.com.* http://www.familyresource.com/lifestyles/mental-environment/television-opiate-of-the-masses, accessed May 29, 2014.

"TV retards your child's development" *Consumers Association of Penang.* http://www.consumer.org.my/index.php/development/education/347-tv-retards-your-childs-development, accessed July 17, 2016.

"Television vs. Reading" *Parent Soup*®, a Trademark of iVillage^sm Inc. Copyright 1996. http://webshare.northseattle.edu/fam180/topics/tv/tvvsread.htm, accessed May 29, 2014.
From Jim Trelease. *The Read-Aloud Handbook*, Penguin Books, 1995.

Thompson, Dennis. "More Americans suffering from stress, anxiety and depression, study finds" *CBS News - Healthday.* http://www.cbsnews.com/news/stress-anxiety-depression-mental-illness-increases-study-finds/, April 17, 2017.

Tintocalis, Ana. "San Francisco Middle Schools No Longer Teaching 'Algebra 1'" *The California Report*, KQED News. http://ww2.kqed.org/news/2015/07/22/san-francisco-middle-schools-no-longer-teaching-algebra-1, July 22, 2015.

Toppo, Greg. "Americans trail adults in other countries in math, literacy, problem-solving" *USA Today.* http://www.usatoday.com/story/news/nation/2013/10/08/literacy-international-workers-education-math-americans/2935909/, October 8, 2013.

Twenge, Jean M.; Thomas E. Joiner; Megan L. Rogers; Gabrielle N. Martin. "Increases in Depressive Symptoms, Suicide-Related Outcomes, and Suicide Rates Among U.S. Adolescents After 2010 and Links to Increased New Media Screen Time" *Clinical Psychological Science.* http://journals.sagepub.com/doi/full/10.1177/2167702617723376, November 14, 2017.

University of Tsukuba. "Active body, active mind: The secret to a younger brain may lie in exercising your body" *ScienceDaily*. http://www.sciencedaily.com/releases/2015/10/151023084456.htm, October 23, 2015.

Van Dyke, Dick. *My Lucky Life*. (New York: Random House, 2011) p. 184.

Vincent van Gogh Gallery. http://www.vggallery.com/, July, 30 2015.

Walter, Tatumn. "A tenth of each day spent watching television (in China)" *USC US-China Institute*. http://www.china.usc.edu/ShowAverageDay.aspx?articleID=2446, accessed May 29, 2014.

"Want a younger brain? Stay in school — and take the stairs" *Science Daily*. https://www.sciencedaily.com/releases/2016/03/160309125520.htm March 9, 2016.

Warner, Jeremy. "Harsh truths about the decline of Britain" *The Telegraph*. http://www.telegraph.co.uk/finance/economics/10417838/Harsh-truths-about-the-decline-of-Britain.html, October 31, 2013.

Washington, Martha. *Letter to Mercy Warren*. 1789. https://en.wikiquote.org/wiki/Martha_Washington.

"What Children are NOT Doing When Watching TV" *American Academy of Pediatrics*. http://www.healthychildren.org/English/family-life/Media/Pages/What-Children-are-NOT-Doing-When-Watching-TV.aspx, May 11, 2013. Original Source: Caring for Your School-Age Child: Ages 5 to 12 (Copyright © 2004 American Academy of Pediatrics).

Williams, Ray. "Anti-Intellectualism and the 'Dumbing Down' of America" *Psychology Today*. https://www.psychologytoday.com/blog/wired-success/201407/anti-intellectualism-and-the-dumbing-down-america. July 7, 2014.

Wilson, Hugh. "Are men becoming more feminine?" *MSN.com*. http://him.uk.msn.com/in-the-know/are-men-becoming-more-feminine-women-male-female-gender-gap, July 19, 2013.

Winn, Marie. *Plug-In Drug* (New York: Viking Penguin, 1977, Revised and Updated Edition, 2002).

Zaki, Jamil. "What, Me Care? Young Are Less Empathetic" A recent study finds a decline in empathy among young people in the U.S. *Scientific American*. http://www.scientificamerican.com/article/what-me-care/, December 23, 2010.

END NOTES

1

- Herbert E. Krugman and Eugene L. Hartley. "Passive Learning From Television" *The Public Opinion Quarterly,* Vol. 34, No. 2. (Oxford University Press, 1970) pp. 184-190.
- Herbert E. Krugman. "Brain Wave Measures of Media Involvement" *How Advertising Works: The Role of Research.* (New York SAGE Publications, 1998) pp. 139–151.
- "Your brain waves change when you watch TV" *I Am Awake.* http://www.iamawake.co/your-brain-waves-change-when-you-watch-tv/, October 11, 2013.
- Allan Stromfeldt Christensen. "Lemminged: to be herded off the peak oil cliff by filmmakers" *TransitionVoice.com.* http://transitionvoice.com/2014/11/lemminged-to-be-herded-off-the-peak-oil-cliff-by-filmmakers/, November 11, 2014.
- "Television: Opiate of the Masses" *FamilyResource.com.* http://www.familyresource.com/lifestyles/mental-environment/television-opiate-of-the-masses, accessed May 29, 2014.
- Douglas Fields. "Watching TV Alters Children's Brain Structure and Lowers IQ". http://rdouglasfields.com/2015/05/watching-tv-alters-childrens-brain-structure-and-lowers-iq/, May 4, 2015.
- Kristina Birdsong. "This is Your Child's Brain on TV" *Scientific Learning.* http://www.scilearn.com/blog/how-television-impacts-learning, Mar 22, 2016.

2

- "TV retards your child's development" *Consumers Association of Penang.* http://www.consumer.org.my/index.php/development/education/347-tv-retards-your-childs-development, accessed July 17, 2016.

- Emma Henderson. "Watching lots of TV 'makes you stupid'" *The Independent.*
  http://www.independent.co.uk/news/science/watching-lots-of-tv-makes-you-stupid-says-american-universities-a6759026.html, December 3, 2015.
- Herbert E. Krugman and Eugene L. Hartley. "Passive Learning From Television" *The Public Opinion Quarterly,* Vol. 34, No. 2. (Oxford University Press, 1970) pp. 184-190.
- Herbert E. Krugman. "Brain Wave Measures of Media Involvement" *How Advertising Works: The Role of Research.* (New York SAGE Publications, 1998) pp. 139–151.
- "Your brain waves change when you watch TV" *I Am Awake.*
  http://www.iamawake.co/your-brain-waves-change-when-you-watch-tv/, October 11, 2013.
- Kristina Birdsong. "This is Your Child's Brain on TV" *Scientific Learning.*
  http://www.scilearn.com/blog/how-television-impacts-learning, Mar 22, 2016.
- Douglas Fields. "Watching TV Alters Children's Brain Structure and Lowers IQ".
  http://rdouglasfields.com/2015/05/watching-tv-alters-childrens-brain-structure-and-lowers-iq/, May 4, 2015.
- Jamil Zaki. "What, Me Care? Young Are Less Empathetic" *Scientific American*. A recent study finds a decline in empathy among young people in the U.S.
  http://www.scientificamerican.com/article/what-me-care/, December 23, 2010.
- "Children who watch 'excessive' amounts of TV are more likely to have criminal convictions, exhibit aggression and experience negative emotions: study." *New York Daily News*.
  http://www.nydailynews.com/life-style/health/kids-watch-excessive-tv-criminal-convictions-young-adulthood-study-article-1.1267868, February 19, 2013.
  "With every hour in front of the television, kids were more likely to show aggressive behavior or receive a criminal conviction by early adulthood, according to a study published in 'Pediatrics.' The issue isn't necessarily the content of the programming, but the social isolation that comes from so many hours in front of the tube."

129

- David L. Hill. "Why to Avoid TV Before Age 2" (early brain development). *American Academy of Pediatrics*. http://www.healthychildren.org/English/family-life/Media/Pages/Why-to-Avoid-TV-Before-Age-2.aspx, May 11, 2013. Original Source: Dad to Dad: Parenting Like a Pro (Copyright © American Academy of Pediatrics 2012).
- Alice Park. "Baby Einsteins: Not So Smart After All" *Time*. http://content.time.com/time/health/article/0,8599,1650352,00.html August 06, 2007.
- "Television vs. Reading" *Parent Soup®*, a Trademark of iVillage[sm] Inc. Copyright 1996. http://webshare.northseattle.edu/fam180/topics/tv/tvvsread.htm, accessed May 29, 2014.
  From Jim Trelease. *The Read-Aloud Handbook*, Penguin Books, 1995.
- Marie Winn. "Television and the Brain" and "Brain Changes" *Plug-In Drug.* (New York: Viking Penguin, 1977, Revised and Updated Edition, 2002) pp. 67–69:
  "'Research conducted during the next two decades removed any doubt about the impact of early brain stimulation on a child's later cognitive development. ... they were able to demonstrate that environmental factors can alter neuron pathways during early childhood and long after ... among the most important of the environmental factors ... are the language and eye contact an infant is exposed to [and] ... the number of words an infant hears each day is the single most important predictor of later intelligence, school success and social competence. But there's one catch. The words have to come from an attentive, engaged human being ... radio and television do not work."

3

- Tom Nichols. *The Death of Expertise.* p. 140. New York: Oxford University Press, 2017.

4

- David Hinckley. "Average American watches 5 hours of TV per day, report shows Time spent watching live TV increases steadily as we get older, according to a new report from Nielsen" *New York Daily News.* http://nydn.us/1fHRJee, Wednesday, March 5, 2014, 5:27 p.m. Per Nielsen, here's the average weekly usage for ascending age groups. Ages:
  - 2–11: 24 hours, 16 minutes. (round down to 24 hours, 15 minutes, or 24.25 x 10 years counting ages 2 and 11 = 12,610)
  - 12–17: 20 hours, 41 minutes. (round down to 20 hours, 30 minutes, or 20.5 hours x 6 years counting ages 12 and 17 = 6,396)
  - 18–24: 22 hours, 27 minutes. (round down to 22 hours, 20 minutes, or 20.33 hours x 6 years counting age 18 to end of age 23 = 6,343)
  - By age 24, the average American has watched 25,349 hours of TV (does not include time on other devices). Here is the breakdown continuing older age groups, showing people watch more and more as they get older. Ages:
    - 25–34: 27 hours, 36 minutes.
    - 35–49: 33 hours, 40 minutes.
    - 50–64: 43 hours, 56 minutes.
    - 65–plus: 50 hours, 34 minutes.
- Victor C. Strasburger, MD, FAAP, and Marjorie J. Hogan, MD, FAAP. "Children, Adolescents, and the Media" *American Academy of Pediatrics.* http://pediatrics.aappublications.org/content/132/5/958.full, May 11, 2013.

5

- Victor C. Strasburger, MD, FAAP, and Marjorie J. Hogan, MD, FAAP. "Children, Adolescents, and the Media". American Academy of Pediatrics. http://pediatrics.aappublications.org/content/132/5/958.full, May 11, 2013.

6

- Alice Park. "Baby Einsteins: Not So Smart After All" *Time.* http://content.time.com/time/health/article/0,8599,1650352,00.html August 06, 2007.

- "Television vs. Reading" *Parent Soup®*, a Trademark of iVillage^{sm} Inc. Copyright 1996. http://webshare.northseattle.edu/fam180/topics/tv/tvvsread.htm, accessed May 29, 2014.
From Jim Trelease. *The Read-Aloud Handbook*, Penguin Books, 1995. Excerpt:

a) Television is the direct opposite of reading. In breaking its programs into eight-minute segments (shorter for shows like Sesame Street), it requires and fosters a short attention span. Reading, on the other hand, requires and encourages longer attention spans. Good children's books are written to hold children's attention, not interrupt it. Because of the need to hold viewers until the next commercial message, the content of television shows is almost constant action. Reading also offers action but not nearly as much, and books fill the spaces between action scenes with subtle character development. Television is relentless; no time is allowed to ponder characters' thoughts or to recall their words because the dialogue and images move too quickly. The need to scrutinize is a critical need among young children, and it is constantly ignored by television. Books, however, encourage the reader to move at his own pace as opposed to that of the director or sponsor. The reader can stop to ponder the character's next move, the feathers in his hat, or the meaning of a sentence. Having done so, he can resume where he left off without having missed any part of the story.

The arrival of remote control is only exacerbating the attention-span problem: the average family "zaps" once every three minutes, twenty-six seconds, versus those who have no remote (once every five minutes, fifteen seconds); and higher-income families zap three times more often than poorer families.

b) For young children television is an antisocial experience, while reading is a social experience. The three-year-old sits passively in front of the screen, oblivious to what is going on around him. Conversation during the program is seldom if ever encouraged by the child or by the parents. On the other hand, the three-year-old with a book must be read to by another person - parent, sibling, or grandparent. The child is a participant as well as a receiver when he engages in discussion during and after the story.

c) Television deprives the child of his most important learning tool: questions. Children learn the most by questioning. For the thirty hours a week that the average five-year-old spends in front of the set, he can neither ask a question nor receive an answer.

d) Television interrupts the child's most important language lesson: family conversation. Studies show the average kindergarten graduate has already seen nearly 6,000 hours of television and videos before entering first grade, hours in which he engaged in little or no conversation. And with 30 percent of all adults watching TV during dinner and 50 percent of preteens and teenagers owning their own sets (and presumably watching alone in their rooms), the description of TV as "the great conversation stopper" has never been more appropriate.

e) Much of young children's television viewing is mindless watching, requiring little or no thinking. When two dozen three-to five-year-olds were shown a Scooby Doo cartoon, the sound track of which had been replaced by the sound track from a Fangface cartoon, only three of the twenty-four children realized the sound track did not match the pictures.

Nor does the mindless viewing stop at kindergarten. With upwards of 100 cable channels to chose from, including all-news stations broadcasting round the clock, one would expect today's young adults to be among the most informed citizens in our history. They are not. A major 1990 survey of 4,890 adults concluded that "young Americans, aged 18 to 30, know less and care less about news and public affairs than any other generation of Americans in the past 50 years." What the X generation absorbs is seldom remembered unless it is titillating. For example, during the Panama invasion, 60 percent said they followed the war closely but only 12 percent were able to identify General Colin Powell. Conversely, 37 percent could identify Donald Trump's alleged mistress, Marla Maples.

f) Television encourages deceptive thinking. In Teaching as a Conserving Activity, Professor Neil Postman pointed out that implicit in every one of television's commercials is the notion that there is no problem that cannot be solved by simple artificial means. Whether the problem is anxiety of common diarrhea, nervous tension or the common cold, a simple tablet or spray solves the problem. Seldom is mention made of headaches being a sign of more serious illness, nor is the suggestion offered that elbow grease and hard work are viable alternatives to stains and boredom. Instead of making us think through our problems, television is enormous when you consider that between ages one and seventeen the average child is exposed to 350,000 commercials (four hundred a week), promoting the idea that solutions to life's problems can be purchased.

g) Television has a negative effect on children's vital knowledge after age ten, according to the Schramm study of 6,000 schoolchildren. It does help, the report goes on to say, in building vocabulary for younger children, but this stops by age ten. This finding is supported by the fact that today's kindergartners have the highest reading-readiness scores ever achieved at that level and yet these same students tail off dismally by fourth and fifth grades. Since television scripts consist largely of conversations that contain the same vocabulary words these students already know, few gains are made.

As I mentioned earlier, shows like Cosby are written on a fourth-grade reading level, hardly an enriching vocabulary for anyone older than eight. Moreover, a study of the scripts from eight programs favored by teenagers showed sentences averaging only seven words (versus eighteen words in my local newspaper). Thus we have the following contrast:
   o   72 percent of the scripts consisted of simple sentences or fragments.
   o   In Make Way for Ducklings, by Robert McCloskey, only 33 percent of the text is simple sentences.

o In *The Tale of Peter Rabbit*, by Beatrix Potter, only 21 percent of the text is simple sentences.
Thus one can safely say that even good children's picture books contain language that is twice as complex as television's. Imagine how much more complex and enriching the novels are.

h) Television stifles the imagination. A study of 192 children from Los Angeles County showed children hearing a story produced more imaginative responses than did those seeing the same story on film.

i) Television's conception of childhood, rather than being progressive, is regressive - a throwback, in fact, to the Middle Ages. Postman points to Philippe Aries's research, which shows that until the 1600s children over the age of five were treated and governed as though they were adults. After the seventeenth century, society developed a concept of childhood which insulated children from the shock of instant adulthood until they were mature enough to meet it. "Television," Postman declares, "all by itself, may bring an end to childhood". I offer these prime examples of that thesis:

In 1991, when children in the Hartford, Connecticut, area saw a network rerun of Peter Pan, they also saw a commercial for an upcoming Hard Copy show about a serial rapist-killer. Repeated incidents like that prompt critics like the Hartford Courant's Jim Endrest to say, "Leaving a child in front of the TV without a parent present is like leaving your kid in the middle of the mall, walking away and hoping he'll find a safe ride home."

The last five years have seen daytime and prime-time television become video encyclopedias for deviant behavior. USA Today columnist Joe Urschel kept notes on one week's representative viewing on such shows. Keep in mind, what you are about to read is only one week's shows, and it was a presidential election week (November 1993). The shows featured: "Aphrodisiacs; Women Who Love Unconditionally; Women Who Killed Their Abusive

135

Husbands; Runaways in Hollywood Who Turn to Prostitution; Possessive Former Lovers; Older Women Who Love Younger Men; Thin Wives, Obese Husbands; Divorcees and Dating; Oft-Married People in Their 20s; Wives and Girlfriends of Mama's Boys; Egotistical Men; Men's Reproductive Rights; The Woman Who Cut Off Her Husband's Penis; Compulsive Gamblers; pre-Menstrual Syndrome; Haunted Houses; Encounters with the Dead; People Who Have Had Encounters with Aliens; Teens Who Kill; Girls in Gangs; Battered Women; Women Who Hate Their Daughters; Murdering Newlyweds; Former Lovers Who Reunite; People Who Stole Their Best Friend's Lover; and Mothers Who Stole Their Daughter's Man." Need I remind you that these shows often were being watched by both parent and child or by a latchkey child alone?

j) Television overpowers and desensitizes a child's sense of sympathy for suffering. Extensive research in the past twenty years clearly shows that television bombardment of the child with continual acts of violence makes the child insensitive to violence and its victims. Any classroom teacher or pediatrician will tell you of the connection between children's viewing of violent films and classroom behavior. From the American Medical Association, June 1994: "Over the past two decades a growing body of scientific research has documented the relationship between the mass media and violent behavior ... namely, that programming shown by the mass media contributes significantly to the aggressive behavior and, in particular, to aggression-related attitudes by many children, adolescents, and adults."

7

- Robert Kubey and Mihaly Csikszentmihalyi. "Television Addiction is no mere metaphor" *Scientific American*. http://www.academia.edu/5065840/Television_Addiction_is_no_mer e_metaphor, accessed January 23, 2016.

8

- "Television: Opiate of the Masses" *FamilyResource.com*. http://www.familyresource.com/lifestyles/mental-environment/television-opiate-of-the-masses, accessed May 29, 2014.

9

- Herbert E. Krugman and Eugene L. Hartley. "Passive Learning From Television" *The Public Opinion Quarterly,* Vol. 34, No. 2. (Oxford University Press, 1970) pp. 184-190.
- Herbert E. Krugman. "Brain Wave Measures of Media Involvement" *How Advertising Works: The Role of Research.* (New York SAGE Publications, 1998) pp. 139–151.
- "Your brain waves change when you watch TV" *I Am Awake.* http://www.iamawake.co/your-brain-waves-change-when-you-watch-tv/, October 11, 2013.

10

- Tom Leonard. "'Passive' TV Can Harm Your Baby's Speech Making It Harder for Them to Later Cope In School" *Daily Mail*. http://www.dailymail.co.uk/news/article-2054950/Passive-TV-watching-harm-babies-speech.html, October 28, 2011.

11

- Kristina Birdsong. "This is Your Child's Brain on TV" *Scientific Learning.* http://www.scilearn.com/blog/how-television-impacts-learning, Mar 22, 2016.

12

- Travis Bradberry and Jean Greaves. *Emotional Intelligence 2.0.* pp. 51, 52. San Diego, California: TalentSmart, 2009.

13

- "TV retards your child's development" *Consumers Association of Penang.* http://www.consumer.org.my/index.php/development/education/347-tv-retards-your-childs-development, accessed July 17, 2016.

- Emma Henderson. "Watching lots of TV 'makes you stupid'" *The Independent.*
  http://www.independent.co.uk/news/science/watching-lots-of-tv-makes-you-stupid-says-american-universities-a6759026.html, December 3, 2015.
- Herbert E. Krugman and Eugene L. Hartley. "Passive Learning From Television" *The Public Opinion Quarterly,* Vol. 34, No. 2. (Oxford University Press, 1970) pp. 184-190.
- Herbert E. Krugman. "Brain Wave Measures of Media Involvement" *How Advertising Works: The Role of Research.* (New York SAGE Publications, 1998) pp. 139–151.
- "Your brain waves change when you watch TV" *I Am Awake.*
  http://www.iamawake.co/your-brain-waves-change-when-you-watch-tv/, October 11, 2013.
- Kristina Birdsong. "This is Your Child's Brain on TV" *Scientific Learning.*
  http://www.scilearn.com/blog/how-television-impacts-learning, Mar 22, 2016.
- Douglas Fields. "Watching TV Alters Children's Brain Structure and Lowers IQ".
  http://rdouglasfields.com/2015/05/watching-tv-alters-childrens-brain-structure-and-lowers-iq/, May 4, 2015.
- Jamil Zaki. "What, Me Care? Young Are Less Empathetic" *Scientific American*. A recent study finds a decline in empathy among young people in the U.S.
  http://www.scientificamerican.com/article/what-me-care/, December 23, 2010.
- "Children who watch 'excessive' amounts of TV are more likely to have criminal convictions, exhibit aggression and experience negative emotions: study." *New York Daily News*.
  http://www.nydailynews.com/life-style/health/kids-watch-excessive-tv-criminal-convictions-young-adulthood-study-article-1.1267868, February 19, 2013.
  "With every hour in front of the television, kids were more likely to show aggressive behavior or receive a criminal conviction by early adulthood, according to a study published in 'Pediatrics.' The issue isn't necessarily the content of the programming, but the social isolation that comes from so many hours in front of the tube."

- David L. Hill. "Why to Avoid TV Before Age 2" (early brain development). *American Academy of Pediatrics*. http://www.healthychildren.org/English/family-life/Media/Pages/Why-to-Avoid-TV-Before-Age-2.aspx, May 11, 2013. Original Source: Dad to Dad: Parenting Like a Pro (Copyright © American Academy of Pediatrics 2012).
- Alice Park. "Baby Einsteins: Not So Smart After All" *Time*. http://content.time.com/time/health/article/0,8599,1650352,00.html August 06, 2007.
- "Television vs. Reading" *Parent Soup*®, a Trademark of iVillage^{sm} Inc. Copyright 1996. http://webshare.northseattle.edu/fam180/topics/tv/tvvsread.htm, accessed May 29, 2014.
  From Jim Trelease. *The Read-Aloud Handbook*, Penguin Books, 1995.
- "What Children are NOT Doing When Watching TV" *American Academy of Pediatrics*. http://www.healthychildren.org/English/family-life/Media/Pages/What-Children-are-NOT-Doing-When-Watching-TV.aspx, May 11, 2013.
  Original Source: *Caring for Your School-Age Child: Ages 5 to 12* (Copyright © 2004 American Academy of Pediatrics).
- Tina D. Hoang, MSPH; Jared Reis, PhD; Na Zhu, MD, MPH; David R. Jacobs Jr, PhD; Lenore J. Launer, PhD; Rachel A. Whitmer, PhD; Stephen Sidney, MD; Kristine Yaffe, MD.
  "Effect of Early Adult Patterns of Physical Activity and Television Viewing on Midlife Cognitive Function" *JAMA Psychiatry* (The Journal of the American Medical Association). http://archpsyc.jamanetwork.com/article.aspx?articleid=2471270, January 2016, Vol 73, No. 1.
- Marie Winn. "Television and the Brain," "Brain Changes," "Losing the Thread," "The Basic Building Blocks," "A Preference for Watching," "Free Time and Resourcefulness" *Plug-In Drug*. (New York: Viking Penguin, 1977, Revised and Updated Edition, 2002) pp. 67–69, 95–99, 131.

14

- Marie Winn. "Losing the Thread," "The Basic Building Blocks," "A Preference for Watching" *Plug-In Drug* (New York: Viking Penguin, 1977, Revised and Updated Edition, 2002) pp. 95–99.
- Herbert E. Krugman and Eugene L. Hartley. "Passive Learning From Television" *The Public Opinion Quarterly,* Vol. 34, No. 2. (Oxford University Press, 1970) pp. 184-190.
- Herbert E. Krugman. "Brain Wave Measures of Media Involvement" *How Advertising Works: The Role of Research.* (New York SAGE Publications, 1998) pp. 139–151.
- "Your brain waves change when you watch TV" *I Am Awake.* http://www.iamawake.co/your-brain-waves-change-when-you-watch-tv/, October 11, 2013.

15

- Kristina Birdsong. "This is Your Child's Brain on TV" *Scientific Learning.* http://www.scilearn.com/blog/how-television-impacts-learning, Mar 22, 2016.

16

- Kristina Birdsong. "This is Your Child's Brain on TV" *Scientific Learning.* http://www.scilearn.com/blog/how-television-impacts-learning, Mar 22, 2016.

17

- Kristina Birdsong. "This is Your Child's Brain on TV" *Scientific Learning.* http://www.scilearn.com/blog/how-television-impacts-learning, Mar 22, 2016.

18

- Marie Winn. "A Commitment to Language" *Plug-In Drug.* (New York: Viking Penguin, 1977, Revised and Updated Edition, 2002) p. 76.
- Alice Park. "Baby Einsteins: Not So Smart After All" *Time.* http://content.time.com/time/health/article/0,8599,1650352,00.htm, August 06, 2007.

19

- David L. Hill. "Why to Avoid TV Before Age 2" (early brain development). *American Academy of Pediatrics*. http://www.healthychildren.org/English/family-life/Media/Pages/Why-to-Avoid-TV-Before-Age-2.aspx, May 11, 2013. Original Source: Dad to Dad: Parenting Like a Pro (Copyright © American Academy of Pediatrics 2012).
- Alice Park. "Baby Einsteins: Not So Smart After All" *Time*. http://content.time.com/time/health/article/0,8599,1650352,00.html August 06, 2007.
- "Television vs. Reading" *Parent Soup*®, a Trademark of iVillage[sm] Inc. Copyright 1996. http://webshare.northseattle.edu/fam180/topics/tv/tvvsread.htm, accessed May 29, 2014.
  From Jim Trelease. *The Read-Aloud Handbook*, Penguin Books, 1995.
- Marie Winn. "Television and the Brain" and "Brain Changes" *Plug-In Drug.* (New York: Viking Penguin, 1977, Revised and Updated Edition, 2002) pp. 67–69:
  "'Research conducted during the next two decades removed any doubt about the impact of early brain stimulation on a child's later cognitive development. … they were able to demonstrate that environmental factors can alter neuron pathways during early childhood and long after … among the most important of the environmental factors … are the language and eye contact an infant is exposed to [and] … the number of words an infant hears each day is the single most important predictor of later intelligence, school success and social competence. But there's one catch. The words have to come from an attentive, engaged human being … radio and television do not work."

20

- Carey Bryson. "Babies and TV: Is Screen Time Good for Your Little One?" *ThoughtCo.* https://www.thoughtco.com/should-babies-watch-tv-2107982, June 22, 2017.

21

- E. Tory Higgins. "Self-Discrepancy Theory" *Advances in Experimental Social Psychology*, Volume 22. Leonard Berkowitz, ed. (Cambridge, Massachusetts: Academic Press. March 28, 1989) p. 119.

22

- E. Tory Higgins. "Self-Discrepancy Theory" *Advances in Experimental Social Psychology*, Volume 22. Leonard Berkowitz, ed. (Cambridge, Massachusetts: Academic Press. March 28, 1989) p. 118.

23

- Nielsen. "Percentage of Americans who say they watch too much TV: 49 %" *BLS American Time Use Survey*, A.C. Nielsen Co. http://www.statisticbrain.com/television-watching-statistics/, Date Verified: 12.7.2013.
- Robert Kubey and Mihaly Csikszentmihalyi "Television Addiction Is No Mere Metaphor" *Scientific American*. http://www.academia.edu/5065840/Television_Addiction_is_no_mere_metaphor, January 23, 2016.

24

- E. Tory Higgins. "Self-Discrepancy Theory" *Advances in Experimental Social Psychology*, Volume 22. Leonard Berkowitz, ed. (Cambridge, Massachusetts: Academic Press. March 28, 1989) p. 118.

25

- Jeff Haden. *The Motivation Myth.* p. 110. New York: Penguin, 2018.

26

- Bob Sornson. "Who's Looking Out for the Children?" *Early Learning Foundation.* http://earlylearningfoundation.com/whos-looking-out-for-the-children/, accessed March 18, 2017.

142

27

- Allan Stromfeldt Christensen. "Lemminged: to be herded off the peak oil cliff by filmmakers" *TransitionVoice.com.* http://transitionvoice.com/2014/11/lemminged-to-be-herded-off-the-peak-oil-cliff-by-filmmakers/, November 11, 2014.

28

- Emma Henderson. "Watching lots of TV 'makes you stupid'" *The Independent.* http://www.independent.co.uk/news/science/watching-lots-of-tv-makes-you-stupid-says-american-universities-a6759026.html, December 3, 2015.
- Tina D. Hoang, MSPH; Jared Reis, PhD; Na Zhu, MD, MPH; David R. Jacobs Jr, PhD; Lenore J. Launer, PhD; Rachel A. Whitmer, PhD; Stephen Sidney, MD; Kristine Yaffe, MD. "Effect of Early Adult Patterns of Physical Activity and Television Viewing on Midlife Cognitive Function" *JAMA Psychiatry* (The Journal of the American Medical Association). http://archpsyc.jamanetwork.com/article.aspx?articleid=2471270, January 2016, Vol 73, No. 1.

29

- Douglas Fields. "Watching TV Alters Children's Brain Structure and Lowers IQ". http://rdouglasfields.com/2015/05/watching-tv-alters-childrens-brain-structure-and-lowers-iq/, May 4, 2015.

30

- Justin Kruger and David Dunning. "Unskilled and Unaware of It: How Difficulties in Recognizing One's Own Incompetence Lead to Inflated Self-Assessments" *Journal of Personality and Social Psychology.* 1999, Vol. 77, No. 6, 1121-1134. Cornell University. http://psych.colorado.edu/~vanboven/teaching/p7536_heurbias/p7536_readings/kruger_dunning.pdf

31

- David Dunning. "We Are All Confident Idiots" *Pacific Standard.* https://www3.nd.edu/~ghaeffel/ConfidentIdiots.pdf, October 27, 2014.

32

- Tom Nichols. *The Death of Expertise.* pp. 119–122, 138. New York: Oxford University Press, 2017.
- Matthew Fisher et al. "Searching for Explanations: How the Internet Inflates Estimates of Internal Knowledge" *Journal of Experimental Psychology* 144(3). pp. 674–687, June 2015.
- Tom Jacobs. "Searching the Internet Creates an Illusion of Knowledge" *Pacific Standard online.* https://psmag.com/environment/searching-internet-creates-the-illusion-of-knowledge-, April 1, 2015.
- Richard Arum. "College Graduates: Satisfied, but Adrift" in *The State of the American Mind.* p. 73, Mark Bauerlein and Adam Bellow, eds. West Conshohocken, PA: Templeton, 2015.

33

- Joe Keohane. "How Facts Backfire: Researchers Discover a Surprising Threat to Democracy: Our Brains" *Boston Globe online.* http://archive.boston.com/bostonglobe/ideas/articles/2010/07/11/how_facts_backfire/, July 11, 2010.
- Tom Nichols. *The Death of Expertise.* p. 131. New York: Oxford University Press, 2017.

34

- Tom Nichols. *The Death of Expertise.* p. 69. New York: Oxford University Press, 2017.

35

- Jessica Stillman. "Which Country Has the Most Productive Workers?" *Inc.com.* http://www.inc.com/jessica-stillman/which-country-has-the-most-productive-workers.html, July 25, 2014.

36

- Jessica Stillman. "The Cold, Hard Truth: You're Overwhelmed Because You Want to Be" *Inc.com.* http://www.inc.com/jessica-stillman/cure-for-feeling-overwhelmed-is-to-stop-talking-about-it.html, March 28, 2014.
- Brigid Schulte. *Overwhelmed: Work, Love, and Play When No One Has the Time.* New York: Simon & Schuster, Inc./Sarah Crichton Books, 2014.

37

- Tatumn Walter. "A tenth of each day spent watching television (in China)" *USC US-China Institute.* http://www.china.usc.edu/ShowAverageDay.aspx?articleID=2446, accessed May 29, 2014.
  This study shows Americans watch 5 hours and 17 minutes a day. Call it 5 hours and 15 minutes (or 5.25 hours / day), and your first 22 years lost 42,157 hours of development time. This study also notes American TV-watching is more than double that of the Chinese.

38

- Travis Bradberry and Jean Greaves. *Emotional Intelligence 2.0.* p. 242. San Diego, California: TalentSmart, 2009.

39

- Jamil Zaki. "What, Me Care? Young Are Less Empathetic" *Scientific American*. A recent study finds a decline in empathy among young people in the U.S. http://www.scientificamerican.com/article/what-me-care/, December 23, 2010.

- "Children who watch 'excessive' amounts of TV are more likely to have criminal convictions, exhibit aggression and experience negative emotions: study." *New York Daily News.* http://www.nydailynews.com/life-style/health/kids-watch-excessive-tv-criminal-convictions-young-adulthood-study-article-1.1267868, February 19, 2013.
  "With every hour in front of the television, kids were more likely to show aggressive behavior or receive a criminal conviction by early adulthood, according to a study published in 'Pediatrics.' The issue isn't necessarily the content of the programming, but the social isolation that comes from so many hours in front of the tube."
- "TV retards your child's development" *Consumers Association of Penang.* http://www.consumer.org.my/index.php/development/education/347-tv-retards-your-childs-development, accessed July 17, 2016.

40

- David Hinckley. "Average American watches 5 hours of TV per day, report shows Time spent watching live TV increases steadily as we get older, according to a new report from Nielsen" *New York Daily News.* http://nydn.us/1fHRJee, Wednesday, March 5, 2014, 5:27 p.m.
  Per Nielsen, here's the average weekly usage for ascending age groups. Ages:
  o 2–11: 24 hours, 16 minutes. (round down to 24 hours, 15 minutes, or 24.25 x 10 years counting ages 2 and 11 = 12,610)
  o 12–17: 20 hours, 41 minutes. (round down to 20 hours, 30 minutes, or 20.5 hours x 6 years counting ages 12 and 17 = 6,396)
  o 18–24: 22 hours, 27 minutes. (round down to 22 hours, 20 minutes, or 20.33 hours x 6 years counting age 18 to end of age 23 = 6,343)
  - By age 24, the average American has watched 25,349 hours of TV (does not include Time on other devices). Here is the breakdown continuing older age groups, showing people watch more and more as they get older. Ages:
    o 25–34: 27 hours, 36 minutes.
    o 35–49: 33 hours, 40 minutes.
    o 50–64: 43 hours, 56 minutes.
    o 65–plus: 50 hours, 34 minutes.

41

- Marie Winn. "Sesame Street Revisited" *Plug-In Drug*. pp. 60, 61. Viking Penguin, 1977, Revised and Updated Edition, 2002.
- Alice Park. "Baby Einsteins: Not So Smart After All" *Time*. http://content.time.com/time/health/article/0,8599,1650352,00.html August 06, 2007.
- *New York Daily News*. Link: http://www.nydailynews.com/life-style/health/kids-watch-excessive-tv-criminal-convictions-young-adulthood-study-article-1.1267868, February 19, 2013. "Children who watch 'excessive' amounts of TV are more likely to have criminal convictions, exhibit aggression and experience negative emotions: study. With every hour in front of the television, kids were more likely to show aggressive behavior or receive a criminal conviction by early adulthood, according to a study published in 'Pediatrics.' The issue isn't necessarily the content of the programming, but the social isolation that comes from so many hours in front of the tube."

42

- "TV retards your child's development" *Consumers Association of Penang*. http://www.consumer.org.my/index.php/development/education/34 7-tv-retards-your-childs-development, accessed July 17, 2016.

43

- Marie Winn. "Sesame Street Revisited" *Plug-In Drug*. pp. 60, 61. Viking Penguin, 1977, Revised and Updated Edition, 2002.
- Alice Park. "Baby Einsteins: Not So Smart After All" *Time*. http://content.time.com/time/health/article/0,8599,1650352,00.html August 06, 2007.
- *New York Daily News*. Link: http://www.nydailynews.com/life-style/health/kids-watch-excessive-tv-criminal-convictions-young-adulthood-study-article-1.1267868, February 19, 2013. "Children who watch 'excessive' amounts of TV are more likely to have criminal convictions, exhibit aggression and experience negative emotions: study. With every hour in front of the television, kids were more likely to show aggressive behavior or receive a criminal

147

conviction by early adulthood, according to a study published in 'Pediatrics.' The issue isn't necessarily the content of the programming, but the social isolation that comes from so many hours in front of the tube."

44

- Herbert E. Krugman and Eugene L. Hartley. "Passive Learning From Television" *The Public Opinion Quarterly,* Vol. 34, No. 2. (Oxford University Press, 1970) pp. 184-190.
- Herbert E. Krugman. "Brain Wave Measures of Media Involvement" *How Advertising Works: The Role of Research.* (New York SAGE Publications, 1998) pp. 139–151.
- "Your brain waves change when you watch TV" *I Am Awake.* http://www.iamawake.co/your-brain-waves-change-when-you-watch-tv/, October 11, 2013.

45

- Tom Nichols. *The Death of Expertise.* p. 69. New York: Oxford University Press, 2017.

46

- Justin Kruger and David Dunning. "Unskilled and Unaware of It: How Difficulties in Recognizing One's Own Incompetence Lead to Inflated Self-Assessments" *Journal of Personality and Social Psychology.* 1999, Vol. 77, No. 6, 1121-1134. Cornell University. http://psych.colorado.edu/~vanboven/teaching/p7536_heurbias/p7536_readings/kruger_dunning.pdf

47

- Allan Stromfeldt Christensen. "Lemminged: to be herded off the peak oil cliff by filmmakers" *TransitionVoice.com.* http://transitionvoice.com/2014/11/lemminged-to-be-herded-off-the-peak-oil-cliff-by-filmmakers/, November 11, 2014.

48

- Robert Kubey and Mihaly Csikszentmihalyi. "Television Addiction is no mere metaphor" *Scientific American.* http://www.academia.edu/5065840/Television_Addiction_is_no_mer e_metaphor, accessed January 23, 2016.

49

- Marie Winn. "Losing the Thread," "The Basic Building Blocks," "A Preference for Watching" *Plug-In Drug.* (New York: Viking Penguin, 1977, Revised and Updated Edition, 2002) pp. 95–99.

50

- Greg Toppo. "Americans trail adults in other countries in math, literacy, problem-solving" *USA Today.*
 "New international study finds U.S. workers lag in math, reading, problem-solving"
 "Adult literacy scores in 12 countries higher than USA, only five score lower"
 http://www.usatoday.com/story/news/nation/2013/10/08/literacy-international-workers-education-math-americans/2935909/, October 8, 2013
- Eric Berger. "By 2010 most science Ph.D.s will go to foreign-born students" *SciGuy.*
 http://blog.chron.com/sciguy/2007/11/by-2010-most-science-ph-d-s-will-go-to-foreign-born-students/, November 21, 2007

51

- Elizabeth Redden. "Foreign Student Dependence" *Inside Higher Education.*
 https://www.insidehighered.com/news/2013/07/12/new-report-shows-dependence-us-graduate-programs-foreign-students, July 12, 2013.

52

- Jane M. Healy. "Endangered Minds" *Creating the Future: Perspectives on Educational Change*. Ed. Dee Dickinson. Johns Hopkins University. 2012. http://education.jhu.edu/PD/newhorizons/future/creating_the_futur e/crfut_healy.cfm

53

- "ISU study finds TV viewing, video game play contribute to kids' attention problems" *Iowa State University*. http://www.news.iastate.edu/news/2010/jul/TVVGattention, July 4, 2010.

54

- Martin Hickman. "Watching TV 'makes toddlers less intelligent'" *The Independent.* http://www.independent.co.uk/news/education/education-news/watching-tv-makes-toddlers-less-intelligent-1960856.html, May 2, 2010.

55

- Josh Constine. "Jeff Bezos' guide to life" *TechCrunch.* https://techcrunch.com/2017/11/05/jeff-bezos-guide-to-life/, November 5, 2017.

56

- Jon Hamilton. "How Play Wires Kids' Brains For Social and Academic Success" *KQED News.* KQED.org, National Public Radio (NPR), Copyright 2014. http://ww2.kqed.org/mindshift/2014/08/07/how-play-wires-kids-brains-for-social-and-academic-success/, August 7, 2014.

57

- Lost development time could be more than 40,000 hours lost in 22 years, counting passive video time on all devices. The number from earlier estimates cited in this book is a conservative 25,349 by age 24. Using other statistics:

- o Nielsen's average hours breakdown for American youth, Americans watch 26,400 hours in their first 22 years.
  Nielsen. BLS American Time Use Survey, A.C. Nielsen Co.
  http://www.statisticbrain.com/television-watching-statistics/, Date Verified: 12.7.2013 (July 12, 2013).
- o Counting 3 devices—TV video, PC-Internet video, mobile-phone video—Average American viewing time is 151 hours per month = 39,864 in 22 years.
  Nielsen. "Television, Internet and Mobile Usage in the U.S. — A2/M2 Three Screen Report 4th Quarter 2008". Copyright © 2009 The Nielsen Company.
  http://i.cdn.turner.com/cnn/2009/images/02/24/screen.press.b.p df, accessed May 29, 2014.
- o Another study shows Americans watch 5 hours and 17 minutes a day. Call it 5 hours and 15 minutes (or 5.25 hours / day), then your first 22 years lost 42,157 hours of development time.
  Tatumn Walter. "A tenth of each day spent watching television (in China)" *USC US-China Institute*.
  http://www.china.usc.edu/ShowAverageDay.aspx?articleID=2446, accessed May 29, 2014.
- o Still another summary of TV studies says "When other screen-based viewing, such as computer games, is included, the figure is far higher. Children aged 11 to 15 now spend 53 hours a week watching TV and computers"
  Aric Sigman. "How TV Is (Quite Literally) Killing Us" *Daily Mail*.
  http://www.whale.to/b/sigman.html, Oct 1, 2005.
- This amount of lost development is leading to more and more video brain-dependency passed along to new generations so that higher brain function will disappear completely.

58

- Victor C. Strasburger, MD, FAAP, and Marjorie J. Hogan, MD, FAAP. "Children, Adolescents, and the Media" *American Academy of Pediatrics*.
  http://pediatrics.aappublications.org/content/132/5/958.full, May 11, 2013.

- "TV retards your child's development" *Consumers Association of Penang.* http://www.consumer.org.my/index.php/development/education/347-tv-retards-your-childs-development, accessed July 17, 2016.
- Emma Henderson. "Watching lots of TV 'makes you stupid'" *The Independent.* http://www.independent.co.uk/news/science/watching-lots-of-tv-makes-you-stupid-says-american-universities-a6759026.html, December 3, 2015.
- Herbert E. Krugman and Eugene L. Hartley. "Passive Learning From Television" *The Public Opinion Quarterly,* Vol. 34, No. 2. (Oxford University Press, 1970) pp. 184-190.
- Herbert E. Krugman. "Brain Wave Measures of Media Involvement" *How Advertising Works: The Role of Research.* (New York SAGE Publications, 1998) pp. 139–151.
- "Your brain waves change when you watch TV" *I Am Awake.* http://www.iamawake.co/your-brain-waves-change-when-you-watch-tv/, October 11, 2013.
- Kristina Birdsong. "This is Your Child's Brain on TV" *Scientific Learning.* http://www.scilearn.com/blog/how-television-impacts-learning, Mar 22, 2016.
- Douglas Fields. "Watching TV Alters Children's Brain Structure and Lowers IQ". http://rdouglasfields.com/2015/05/watching-tv-alters-childrens-brain-structure-and-lowers-iq/, May 4, 2015.
- Jamil Zaki. "What, Me Care? Young Are Less Empathetic" *Scientific American.* A recent study finds a decline in empathy among young people in the U.S. http://www.scientificamerican.com/article/what-me-care/, December 23, 2010.
- "Children who watch 'excessive' amounts of TV are more likely to have criminal convictions, exhibit aggression and experience negative emotions: study." *New York Daily News.* http://www.nydailynews.com/life-style/health/kids-watch-excessive-tv-criminal-convictions-young-adulthood-study-article-1.1267868, February 19, 2013.

"With every hour in front of the television, kids were more likely to show aggressive behavior or receive a criminal conviction by early adulthood, according to a study published in 'Pediatrics.' The issue isn't necessarily the content of the programming, but the social isolation that comes from so many hours in front of the tube."

- David L. Hill. "Why to Avoid TV Before Age 2" (early brain development). *American Academy of Pediatrics*. http://www.healthychildren.org/English/family-life/Media/Pages/Why-to-Avoid-TV-Before-Age-2.aspx, May 11, 2013. Original Source: Dad to Dad: Parenting Like a Pro (Copyright © American Academy of Pediatrics 2012).
- Alice Park. "Baby Einsteins: Not So Smart After All" *Time*. http://content.time.com/time/health/article/0,8599,1650352,00.html August 06, 2007.
- "Television vs. Reading" *Parent Soup*®, a Trademark of iVillage[sm] Inc. Copyright 1996. http://webshare.northseattle.edu/fam180/topics/tv/tvvsread.htm, accessed May 29, 2014. From Jim Trelease. *The Read-Aloud Handbook*, Penguin Books, 1995.
- "What Children are NOT Doing When Watching TV" *American Academy of Pediatrics*. http://www.healthychildren.org/English/family-life/Media/Pages/What-Children-are-NOT-Doing-When-Watching-TV.aspx, May 11, 2013. Original Source: *Caring for Your School-Age Child: Ages 5 to 12* (Copyright © 2004 American Academy of Pediatrics).
- Tina D. Hoang, MSPH; Jared Reis, PhD; Na Zhu, MD, MPH; David R. Jacobs Jr, PhD; Lenore J. Launer, PhD; Rachel A. Whitmer, PhD; Stephen Sidney, MD; Kristine Yaffe, MD. "Effect of Early Adult Patterns of Physical Activity and Television Viewing on Midlife Cognitive Function" *JAMA Psychiatry* (The Journal of the American Medical Association). http://archpsyc.jamanetwork.com/article.aspx?articleid=2471270, January 2016, Vol 73, No. 1.
- Marie Winn. "Television and the Brain," "Brain Changes," "Losing the Thread," "The Basic Building Blocks," "A Preference for Watching," "Free Time and Resourcefulness" *Plug-In Drug*. (New York: Viking

Penguin, 1977, Revised and Updated Edition, 2002) pp. 67–69, 95–99, 131.

60

- Kristina Birdsong. "This is Your Child's Brain on TV" *Scientific Learning.* http://www.scilearn.com/blog/how-television-impacts-learning, Mar 22, 2016.

61

- Robert Kubey and Mihaly Csikszentmihalyi. "Television Addiction is no mere metaphor" *Scientific American.* http://www.academia.edu/5065840/Television_Addiction_is_no_mer e_metaphor, accessed January 23, 2016.

62

- Bruno S. Frey, Christine Benesch, Alois Stutzer. "Does watching TV make us happy?" *Journal of Economic Psychology*, Volume 28, Issue 3, June 2007. Elsevier B.V. (ScienceDirect.com). http://www.bsfrey.ch/articles/459_07.pdf, February 14, 2007.

63

- Robert Kubey and Mihaly Csikszentmihalyi. "Television Addiction is no mere metaphor" *Scientific American.* http://www.academia.edu/5065840/Television_Addiction_is_no_mer e_metaphor, accessed January 23, 2016.

64

- Jim Taylor. "Pro Athletes are Hooked on Social Media Too". http://www.drjimtaylor.com/4.0/pro-athletes-are-hooked-on-social-media-too/, accessed April 23, 2018.
- Candace Buckner. "NBA players know they're addicted to their phones. Good luck getting them to unplug" *The Washington Post.* https://www.washingtonpost.com/sports/nba-players-know-theyre-addicted-to-their-phones-good-luck-getting-them-to-unplug/2018/03/19/6165cb96-2563-11e8-b79d-f3d931db7f68_story.html, March 19, 2018.

65

- Marie Winn. "A Chilling Episode: The 'Tired-Child Syndrome'" *Plug-In Drug.* (New York: Viking Penguin, 1977, Revised and Updated Edition, 2002) p.219, 220.

66

- Marie Winn. "A Chilling Episode: The 'Tired-Child Syndrome'" *Plug-In Drug.* (New York: Viking Penguin, 1977, Revised and Updated Edition, 2002) p.219, 220.

67

- Adam Alter. "Tech Bigwigs Know How Addictive Their Products Are. Why Don't the Rest of Us?" *Wired.com.* https://www.wired.com/2017/03/irresistible-the-rise-of-addictive-technology-and-the-business-of-keeping-us-hooked/, March 24, 2017.

68

- Adam Alter. "Tech Bigwigs Know How Addictive Their Products Are. Why Don't the Rest of Us?" *Wired.com.* https://www.wired.com/2017/03/irresistible-the-rise-of-addictive-technology-and-the-business-of-keeping-us-hooked/, March 24, 2017.

69

- Adam Alter. "Tech Bigwigs Know How Addictive Their Products Are. Why Don't the Rest of Us?" *Wired.com.* https://www.wired.com/2017/03/irresistible-the-rise-of-addictive-technology-and-the-business-of-keeping-us-hooked/, March 24, 2017.

70

- Adam Alter. "Tech Bigwigs Know How Addictive Their Products Are. Why Don't the Rest of Us?" *Wired.com.* https://www.wired.com/2017/03/irresistible-the-rise-of-addictive-technology-and-the-business-of-keeping-us-hooked/, March 24, 2017.

71

- Adam Alter. "Tech Bigwigs Know How Addictive Their Products Are. Why Don't the Rest of Us?" *Wired.com*. https://www.wired.com/2017/03/irresistible-the-rise-of-addictive-technology-and-the-business-of-keeping-us-hooked/, March 24, 2017.

72

- Adam Alter. "Tech Bigwigs Know How Addictive Their Products Are. Why Don't the Rest of Us?" *Wired.com*. https://www.wired.com/2017/03/irresistible-the-rise-of-addictive-technology-and-the-business-of-keeping-us-hooked/, March 24, 2017.

73

- Jean M. Twenge, Thomas E. Joiner, Megan L. Rogers, Gabrielle N. Martin. "Increases in Depressive Symptoms, Suicide-Related Outcomes, and Suicide Rates Among U.S. Adolescents After 2010 and Links to Increased New Media Screen Time" *Clinical Psychological Science*. http://journals.sagepub.com/doi/full/10.1177/2167702617723376, November 14, 2017.

74

- Jean M. Twenge, Thomas E. Joiner, Megan L. Rogers, Gabrielle N. Martin. "Increases in Depressive Symptoms, Suicide-Related Outcomes, and Suicide Rates Among U.S. Adolescents After 2010 and Links to Increased New Media Screen Time" *Clinical Psychological Science*. http://journals.sagepub.com/doi/full/10.1177/2167702617723376, November 14, 2017.

75

- Jean M. Twenge, Thomas E. Joiner, Megan L. Rogers, Gabrielle N. Martin. "Increases in Depressive Symptoms, Suicide-Related Outcomes, and Suicide Rates Among U.S. Adolescents After 2010 and Links to Increased New Media Screen Time" *Clinical Psychological Science*. http://journals.sagepub.com/doi/full/10.1177/2167702617723376, November 14, 2017.

76

- Jean M. Twenge, Thomas E. Joiner, Megan L. Rogers, Gabrielle N. Martin. "Increases in Depressive Symptoms, Suicide-Related Outcomes, and Suicide Rates Among U.S. Adolescents After 2010 and Links to Increased New Media Screen Time" *Clinical Psychological Science.* http://journals.sagepub.com/doi/full/10.1177/2167702617723376, November 14, 2017.
"iGen" Note: "The generations represented here include GenX (born approximately 1965–1979), Millennials (1980–1994), and iGen (1995–2012)" (Twenge).

- To help with generations that are mentioned, here is a table showing the birth years for seven generations, most recent on top:

Birth Date	Generation Label
1996 to 2015	Centennials, iGeneration (iGen) or Generation Z (GenZ)
1977 to 1995	Millennials or Generation Y (GenY)
1965 to 1976	Generation X (GenX)
1946 to 1964	Baby Boomers
1926 to 1945	Traditionalists or Silent Generation
1901 to 1925	G.I. Generation or World War II Generation
1883 to 1900	Lost Generation, Generation of 1914 or World War I Generation

77

- Jeff Haden. *The Motivation Myth.* p. 211. New York: Penguin, 2018.

78

- Elise Hu. "Facebook Makes Us Sadder And Less Satisfied, Study Finds" *National Public Radio.* http://www.npr.org/blogs/alltechconsidered/2013/08/19/213568763/researchers-facebook-makes-us-sadder-and-less-satisfied, August 20, 2013.
  "If you're feeling bummed, researchers did test for and find a solution. The prescription for Facebook despair is less Facebook. Researchers found that face-to-face or phone interaction — those outmoded, analog ways of communication — had the opposite effect. Direct interactions with other human beings led people to feel better."

79

- Adam Alter. "Tech Bigwigs Know How Addictive Their Products Are. Why Don't the Rest of Us?" *Wired.com.* https://www.wired.com/2017/03/irresistible-the-rise-of-addictive-technology-and-the-business-of-keeping-us-hooked/, March 24, 2017.

80

- Eric Pickersgill. *Removed.* http://www.removed.social/, accessed October 21, 2015.

81

- Ethan Kross, Philippe Verduyn, Emre Demiralp, Jiyoung Park, David Seungjae Lee, Natalie Lin, Holly Shablack, John Jonides, Oscar Ybarra. "Facebook Use Predicts Declines in Subjective Well-Being in Young Adults" *PLoS ONE* 8(8): e69841. doi:10.1371/journal.pone.0069841. http://www.plosone.org/article/info%3Adoi%2F10.1371%2Fjournal.pone.0069841, August 14, 2013.

82

- Dennis Thompson. "More Americans suffering from stress, anxiety and depression, study finds" *CBS News - Healthday.* http://www.cbsnews.com/news/stress-anxiety-depression-mental-illness-increases-study-finds/, April 17, 2017.

- Mel Schwartz. "Is Our Society Manufacturing Depressed People?" *Psychology Today.* https://www.psychologytoday.com/blog/shift-mind/201203/is-our-society-manufacturing-depressed-people, March 19, 2012.

83

- Jean M. Twenge, Thomas E. Joiner, Megan L. Rogers, Gabrielle N. Martin. "Increases in Depressive Symptoms, Suicide-Related Outcomes, and Suicide Rates Among U.S. Adolescents After 2010 and Links to Increased New Media Screen Time" *Clinical Psychological Science.* http://journals.sagepub.com/doi/full/10.1177/2167702617723376, November 14, 2017.

84

- Dennis Thompson. "More Americans suffering from stress, anxiety and depression, study finds" *CBS News - Healthday.* http://www.cbsnews.com/news/stress-anxiety-depression-mental-illness-increases-study-finds/, April 17, 2017.

85

- Travis Bradberry. "13 Habits of Exceptionally Likeable People". https://www.linkedin.com/pulse/13-habits-exceptionally-likeable-people-dr-travis-bradberry, January 27, 2015.

86

- Jean M. Twenge, Thomas E. Joiner, Megan L. Rogers, Gabrielle N. Martin. "Increases in Depressive Symptoms, Suicide-Related Outcomes, and Suicide Rates Among U.S. Adolescents After 2010 and Links to Increased New Media Screen Time" *Clinical Psychological Science.* http://journals.sagepub.com/doi/full/10.1177/2167702617723376, November 14, 2017.

87

- Jamil Zaki. "What, Me Care? Young Are Less Empathetic" *Scientific American*. A recent study finds a decline in empathy among young people in the U.S.
http://www.scientificamerican.com/article/what-me-care/,
December 23, 2010.
- "Children who watch 'excessive' amounts of TV are more likely to have criminal convictions, exhibit aggression and experience negative emotions: study." *New York Daily News*.
http://www.nydailynews.com/life-style/health/kids-watch-excessive-tv-criminal-convictions-young-adulthood-study-article-1.1267868,
February 19, 2013.
"With every hour in front of the television, kids were more likely to show aggressive behavior or receive a criminal conviction by early adulthood, according to a study published in 'Pediatrics.' The issue isn't necessarily the content of the programming, but the social isolation that comes from so many hours in front of the tube."
- "TV retards your child's development" *Consumers Association of Penang.*
http://www.consumer.org.my/index.php/development/education/34
7-tv-retards-your-childs-development, accessed July 17, 2016.
- Emma Henderson. "Watching lots of TV 'makes you stupid'" *The Independent.*
http://www.independent.co.uk/news/science/watching-lots-of-tv-makes-you-stupid-says-american-universities-a6759026.html,
December 3, 2015.
- Herbert E. Krugman and Eugene L. Hartley. "Passive Learning From Television" *The Public Opinion Quarterly,* Vol. 34, No. 2. (Oxford University Press, 1970) pp. 184-190.
- Herbert E. Krugman. "Brain Wave Measures of Media Involvement" *How Advertising Works: The Role of Research.* (New York SAGE Publications, 1998) pp. 139–151.
- "Your brain waves change when you watch TV" *I Am Awake.*
http://www.iamawake.co/your-brain-waves-change-when-you-watch-tv/, October 11, 2013.

- Kristina Birdsong. "This is Your Child's Brain on TV" *Scientific Learning.* http://www.scilearn.com/blog/how-television-impacts-learning, Mar 22, 2016.
- Douglas Fields. "Watching TV Alters Children's Brain Structure and Lowers IQ". http://rdouglasfields.com/2015/05/watching-tv-alters-childrens-brain-structure-and-lowers-iq/, May 4, 2015.
- David L. Hill. "Why to Avoid TV Before Age 2" (early brain development). *American Academy of Pediatrics*. http://www.healthychildren.org/English/family-life/Media/Pages/Why-to-Avoid-TV-Before-Age-2.aspx, May 11, 2013. Original Source: Dad to Dad: Parenting Like a Pro (Copyright © American Academy of Pediatrics 2012).
- Alice Park. "Baby Einsteins: Not So Smart After All" *Time*. http://content.time.com/time/health/article/0,8599,1650352,00.html August 06, 2007.
- "Television vs. Reading" *Parent Soup*®, a Trademark of iVillage^sm Inc. Copyright 1996. http://webshare.northseattle.edu/fam180/topics/tv/tvvsread.htm, accessed May 29, 2014.
  From Jim Trelease. *The Read-Aloud Handbook*, Penguin Books, 1995.
- Marie Winn. "Television and the Brain" and "Brain Changes" *Plug-In Drug.* (New York: Viking Penguin, 1977, Revised and Updated Edition, 2002) pp. 67–69:
  "'Research conducted during the next two decades removed any doubt about the impact of early brain stimulation on a child's later cognitive development. … they were able to demonstrate that environmental factors can alter neuron pathways during early childhood and long after … among the most important of the environmental factors … are the language and eye contact an infant is exposed to [and] … the number of words an infant hears each day is the single most important predictor of later intelligence, school success and social competence. But there's one catch. The words have to come from an attentive, engaged human being … radio and television do not work."

88

- Maia Szalavitz. "Misery Has More Company Than You Think, Especially on Facebook" *Time*. http://healthland.time.com/2011/01/27/youre-not-alone-misery-has-more-company-than-you-think/, January 27, 2011.
- Alexander H. Jordan, Benoît Monin, Carol S. Dweck, Benjamin J. Lovett, Oliver P. John, and James J. Gross. "Misery Has More Company Than People Think: Underestimating the Prevalence of Others' Negative Emotions" *Personality and Social Psychology Bulletin* January 2011 37: 120-135. National Institutes of Health. http://www.ncbi.nlm.nih.gov/pmc/articles/PMC4138214/, January 2011, latest update August 19, 2014.
- Elise Hu. "Facebook Makes Us Sadder And Less Satisfied, Study Finds" *National Public Radio*. http://www.npr.org/blogs/alltechconsidered/2013/08/19/213568763/researchers-facebook-makes-us-sadder-and-less-satisfied, August 20, 2013.
  "If you're feeling bummed, researchers did test for and find a solution. The prescription for Facebook despair is less Facebook. Researchers found that face-to-face or phone interaction — those outmoded, analog ways of communication — had the opposite effect. Direct interactions with other human beings led people to feel better."
- Ethan Kross, Philippe Verduyn, Emre Demiralp, Jiyoung Park, David Seungjae Lee, Natalie Lin, Holly Shablack, John Jonides, Oscar Ybarra. "Facebook Use Predicts Declines in Subjective Well-Being in Young Adults" *PLoS ONE* 8(8): e69841. doi:10.1371/journal.pone.0069841. http://www.plosone.org/article/info%3Adoi%2F10.1371%2Fjournal.pone.0069841, August 14, 2013.

89

- Herbert E. Krugman and Eugene L. Hartley. "Passive Learning From Television" *The Public Opinion Quarterly,* Vol. 34, No. 2. (Oxford University Press, 1970) pp. 184-190.
- Herbert E. Krugman. "Brain Wave Measures of Media Involvement" *How Advertising Works: The Role of Research.* (New York SAGE Publications, 1998) pp. 139–151.

- "Your brain waves change when you watch TV" *I Am Awake.* http://www.iamawake.co/your-brain-waves-change-when-you-watch-tv/, October 11, 2013.

90

- Jean M. Twenge, Thomas E. Joiner, Megan L. Rogers, Gabrielle N. Martin. "Increases in Depressive Symptoms, Suicide-Related Outcomes, and Suicide Rates Among U.S. Adolescents After 2010 and Links to Increased New Media Screen Time" *Clinical Psychological Science.* http://journals.sagepub.com/doi/full/10.1177/2167702617723376, November 14, 2017.

91

- Robert Kubey and Mihaly Csikszentmihalyi. "Television Addiction is no mere metaphor" *Scientific American.* http://www.academia.edu/5065840/Television_Addiction_is_no_mer e_metaphor, accessed January 23, 2016.

92

- Marie Winn. "Losing the Thread," "The Basic Building Blocks," "A Preference for Watching" *Plug-In Drug.* (New York: Viking Penguin, 1977, Revised and Updated Edition, 2002) pp. 95–99.

93

- Robert Kubey and Mihaly Csikszentmihalyi. "Television Addiction is no mere metaphor" *Scientific American.* http://www.academia.edu/5065840/Television_Addiction_is_no_mer e_metaphor, accessed January 23, 2016.

94

- Robert Kubey and Mihaly Csikszentmihalyi. "Television Addiction is no mere metaphor" *Scientific American.* http://www.academia.edu/5065840/Television_Addiction_is_no_mer e_metaphor, accessed January 23, 2016.

95

- Jessica Stillman. "The Cold, Hard Truth: You're Overwhelmed Because You Want to Be" *Inc.com.* http://www.inc.com/jessica-stillman/cure-for-feeling-overwhelmed-is-to-stop-talking-about-it.html, March 28, 2014.

96

- Jessica Stillman. "The Cold, Hard Truth: You're Overwhelmed Because You Want to Be" *Inc.com.* http://www.inc.com/jessica-stillman/cure-for-feeling-overwhelmed-is-to-stop-talking-about-it.html, March 28, 2014.

97

- Jessica Stillman. "Complaining Is Terrible for You, According to Science". *Inc.com.* http://www.inc.com/jessica-stillman/complaining-rewires-your-brain-for-negativity-science-says.html, February 29, 2016.

98

- William F. Doverspike, Ph.D. "How To Make Yourself Miserable: Discovering the Secrets to Unhappiness" *Georgia Psychological Association*. Atlanta. http://gapsychology.org/displaycommon.cfm?an=1&subarticlenbr=341, accessed September 29, 2014.
- Belinda Goldsmith. "Watching hours of TV daily could shorten your life – study" Ed. Miral Fahmy. *Reuters*. http://in.reuters.com/article/worldNews/idINIndia-45316820100111, January 12, 2010.

99

- Travis Bradberry. "13 Things Mentally Strong People Won't Do". https://www.linkedin.com/pulse/13-things-mentally-strong-people-wont-do-dr-travis-bradberry/, September 11, 2017.

100

- Maya Angelou, quoted in *Maya Angelou: 365 Quotes and Sayings of Phenomenal Woman*, by Maura Craig. (quote #348). Sep 27, 2014. Google digitized version: https://books.google.com/books?id=UKiiBAAAQBAJ&pg=PT73.

101

- William F. Doverspike, Ph.D. "How To Make Yourself Miserable: Discovering the Secrets to Unhappiness" *Georgia Psychological Association*. Atlanta. http://gapsychology.org/displaycommon.cfm?an=1&subarticlenbr=341, accessed September 29, 2014.

102

- "TV retards your child's development" *Consumers Association of Penang.* http://www.consumer.org.my/index.php/development/education/347-tv-retards-your-childs-development, accessed July 17, 2016.
- Emma Henderson. "Watching lots of TV 'makes you stupid'" *The Independent.* http://www.independent.co.uk/news/science/watching-lots-of-tv-makes-you-stupid-says-american-universities-a6759026.html, December 3, 2015.
- Herbert E. Krugman and Eugene L. Hartley. "Passive Learning From Television" *The Public Opinion Quarterly,* Vol. 34, No. 2. (Oxford University Press, 1970) pp. 184-190.
- Herbert E. Krugman. "Brain Wave Measures of Media Involvement" *How Advertising Works: The Role of Research.* (New York SAGE Publications, 1998) pp. 139–151.
- "Your brain waves change when you watch TV" *I Am Awake.* http://www.iamawake.co/your-brain-waves-change-when-you-watch-tv/, October 11, 2013.
- Kristina Birdsong. "This is Your Child's Brain on TV" *Scientific Learning.* http://www.scilearn.com/blog/how-television-impacts-learning, Mar 22, 2016.
- Douglas Fields. "Watching TV Alters Children's Brain Structure and Lowers IQ".

http://rdouglasfields.com/2015/05/watching-tv-alters-childrens-brain-structure-and-lowers-iq/, May 4, 2015.

- Jamil Zaki. "What, Me Care? Young Are Less Empathetic" *Scientific American*. A recent study finds a decline in empathy among young people in the U.S.
http://www.scientificamerican.com/article/what-me-care/, December 23, 2010.

- "Children who watch 'excessive' amounts of TV are more likely to have criminal convictions, exhibit aggression and experience negative emotions: study." *New York Daily News*.
http://www.nydailynews.com/life-style/health/kids-watch-excessive-tv-criminal-convictions-young-adulthood-study-article-1.1267868, February 19, 2013.
"With every hour in front of the television, kids were more likely to show aggressive behavior or receive a criminal conviction by early adulthood, according to a study published in 'Pediatrics.' The issue isn't necessarily the content of the programming, but the social isolation that comes from so many hours in front of the tube."

- David L. Hill. "Why to Avoid TV Before Age 2" (early brain development). *American Academy of Pediatrics*.
http://www.healthychildren.org/English/family-life/Media/Pages/Why-to-Avoid-TV-Before-Age-2.aspx, May 11, 2013.
Original Source: Dad to Dad: Parenting Like a Pro (Copyright © American Academy of Pediatrics 2012).

- Alice Park. "Baby Einsteins: Not So Smart After All" *Time*.
http://content.time.com/time/health/article/0,8599,1650352,00.html August 06, 2007.

- "Television vs. Reading" *Parent Soup®*, a Trademark of iVillage℠ Inc. Copyright 1996.
http://webshare.northseattle.edu/fam180/topics/tv/tvvsread.htm, accessed May 29, 2014.
From Jim Trelease. *The Read-Aloud Handbook*, Penguin Books, 1995.

- "What Children are NOT Doing When Watching TV" *American Academy of Pediatrics*.
http://www.healthychildren.org/English/family-life/Media/Pages/What-Children-are-NOT-Doing-When-Watching-TV.aspx, May 11, 2013.

Original Source: *Caring for Your School-Age Child: Ages 5 to 12* (Copyright © 2004 American Academy of Pediatrics).

- Tina D. Hoang, MSPH; Jared Reis, PhD; Na Zhu, MD, MPH; David R. Jacobs Jr, PhD; Lenore J. Launer, PhD; Rachel A. Whitmer, PhD; Stephen Sidney, MD; Kristine Yaffe, MD.
  "Effect of Early Adult Patterns of Physical Activity and Television Viewing on Midlife Cognitive Function" *JAMA Psychiatry* (The Journal of the American Medical Association).
  http://archpsyc.jamanetwork.com/article.aspx?articleid=2471270, January 2016, Vol 73, No. 1.

- Marie Winn. "Television and the Brain," "Brain Changes," "Losing the Thread," "The Basic Building Blocks," "A Preference for Watching," "Free Time and Resourcefulness" *Plug-In Drug.* (New York: Viking Penguin, 1977, Revised and Updated Edition, 2002) pp. 67–69, 95–99, 131.

103

- Allan Stromfeldt Christensen. "Lemminged: to be herded off the peak oil cliff by filmmakers" *TransitionVoice.com.*
  http://transitionvoice.com/2014/11/lemminged-to-be-herded-off-the-peak-oil-cliff-by-filmmakers/, November 11, 2014.

104

- Allan Stromfeldt Christensen. "Lemminged: to be herded off the peak oil cliff by filmmakers" *TransitionVoice.com.*
  http://transitionvoice.com/2014/11/lemminged-to-be-herded-off-the-peak-oil-cliff-by-filmmakers/, November 11, 2014.

105

- Allan Stromfeldt Christensen. "Lemminged: to be herded off the peak oil cliff by filmmakers" *TransitionVoice.com.*
  http://transitionvoice.com/2014/11/lemminged-to-be-herded-off-the-peak-oil-cliff-by-filmmakers/, November 11, 2014.

106

- Allan Stromfeldt Christensen. "Lemminged: to be herded off the peak oil cliff by filmmakers" *TransitionVoice.com*. http://transitionvoice.com/2014/11/lemminged-to-be-herded-off-the-peak-oil-cliff-by-filmmakers/, November 11, 2014.

107

- Allan Stromfeldt Christensen. "Lemminged: to be herded off the peak oil cliff by filmmakers" *TransitionVoice.com*. http://transitionvoice.com/2014/11/lemminged-to-be-herded-off-the-peak-oil-cliff-by-filmmakers/, November 11, 2014.

108

- "Planet or Plastic? A Brief History of How Plastic Has Changed Our World" *National Geographic*. https://video.nationalgeographic.com/video/magazine/planet-or-plastic/180516-ngm-brief-history-of-plastic, Accessed May 18, 2018.

109

- Allan Stromfeldt Christensen. "Lemminged: to be herded off the peak oil cliff by filmmakers" *TransitionVoice.com*. http://transitionvoice.com/2014/11/lemminged-to-be-herded-off-the-peak-oil-cliff-by-filmmakers/, November 11, 2014.

110

- Eric Holthaus and Chris Kirk. "A Filthy History: Interactive map: Which countries have emitted the most carbon since 1850?" *Slate.com*. http://www.slate.com/articles/technology/future_tense/2014/05/carbon_dioxide_emissions_by_country_over_time_the_worst_global_warming_polluters.html.

111

- "Carbon footprint" *Wikipedia*. http://en.wikipedia.org/wiki/Carbon_footprint, accessed November 1, 2014.

112

- Eric Holthaus and Chris Kirk. "A Filthy History: Interactive map: Which countries have emitted the most carbon since 1850?" *Slate.com.* http://www.slate.com/articles/technology/future_tense/2014/05/carbon_dioxide_emissions_by_country_over_time_the_worst_global_warming_polluters.html.

113

- "How Satellites Work With Mobile Phones" *CompareMyMobile.* http://blog.comparemymobile.com/how-satellites-work-with-mobile-phones/, accessed December 21, 2017.

114

- Sharon Jayson. "Generation Y's goal? Wealth and fame" *USA Today.* http://usatoday30.usatoday.com/news/nation/2007-01-09-gen-y-cover_x.htm, Posted January 9,2007, Updated January 10, 2007.

115

- "TV retards your child's development" *Consumers Association of Penang.* http://www.consumer.org.my/index.php/development/education/347-tv-retards-your-childs-development, accessed July 17, 2016.
- Emma Henderson. "Watching lots of TV 'makes you stupid'" *The Independent.* http://www.independent.co.uk/news/science/watching-lots-of-tv-makes-you-stupid-says-american-universities-a6759026.html, December 3, 2015.
- Herbert E. Krugman and Eugene L. Hartley. "Passive Learning From Television" *The Public Opinion Quarterly,* Vol. 34, No. 2. (Oxford University Press, 1970) pp. 184-190.
- Herbert E. Krugman. "Brain Wave Measures of Media Involvement" *How Advertising Works: The Role of Research.* (New York SAGE Publications, 1998) pp. 139–151.
- "Your brain waves change when you watch TV" *I Am Awake.* http://www.iamawake.co/your-brain-waves-change-when-you-watch-tv/, October 11, 2013.

- Kristina Birdsong. "This is Your Child's Brain on TV" *Scientific Learning.* http://www.scilearn.com/blog/how-television-impacts-learning, Mar 22, 2016.
- Douglas Fields. "Watching TV Alters Children's Brain Structure and Lowers IQ". http://rdouglasfields.com/2015/05/watching-tv-alters-childrens-brain-structure-and-lowers-iq/, May 4, 2015.
- Jamil Zaki. "What, Me Care? Young Are Less Empathetic" *Scientific American*. A recent study finds a decline in empathy among young people in the U.S. http://www.scientificamerican.com/article/what-me-care/, December 23, 2010.
- "Children who watch 'excessive' amounts of TV are more likely to have criminal convictions, exhibit aggression and experience negative emotions: study." *New York Daily News*. http://www.nydailynews.com/life-style/health/kids-watch-excessive-tv-criminal-convictions-young-adulthood-study-article-1.1267868, February 19, 2013.
  "With every hour in front of the television, kids were more likely to show aggressive behavior or receive a criminal conviction by early adulthood, according to a study published in 'Pediatrics.' The issue isn't necessarily the content of the programming, but the social isolation that comes from so many hours in front of the tube."
- David L. Hill. "Why to Avoid TV Before Age 2" (early brain development). *American Academy of Pediatrics*. http://www.healthychildren.org/English/family-life/Media/Pages/Why-to-Avoid-TV-Before-Age-2.aspx, May 11, 2013. Original Source: Dad to Dad: Parenting Like a Pro (Copyright © American Academy of Pediatrics 2012).
- Alice Park. "Baby Einsteins: Not So Smart After All" *Time*. http://content.time.com/time/health/article/0,8599,1650352,00.html August 06, 2007.
- "Television vs. Reading" *Parent Soup*®, a Trademark of iVillage℠ Inc. Copyright 1996. http://webshare.northseattle.edu/fam180/topics/tv/tvvsread.htm, accessed May 29, 2014.
  From Jim Trelease. *The Read-Aloud Handbook*, Penguin Books, 1995.

- Marie Winn. "Television and the Brain" and "Brain Changes" *Plug-In Drug.* (New York: Viking Penguin, 1977, Revised and Updated Edition, 2002) pp. 67–69:
  "'Research conducted during the next two decades removed any doubt about the impact of early brain stimulation on a child's later cognitive development. ... they were able to demonstrate that environmental factors can alter neuron pathways during early childhood and long after ... among the most important of the environmental factors ... are the language and eye contact an infant is exposed to [and] ... the number of words an infant hears each day is the single most important predictor of later intelligence, school success and social competence. But there's one catch. The words have to come from an attentive, engaged human being ... radio and television do not work."

116

- Marie Winn. "Losing the Thread," "The Basic Building Blocks," "A Preference for Watching" *Plug-In Drug.* (New York: Viking Penguin, 1977, Revised and Updated Edition, 2002) pp. 95–99.

117

- Robert Kubey and Mihaly Csikszentmihalyi. "Television Addiction is no mere metaphor" Scientific American.
  http://www.academia.edu/5065840/Television_Addiction_is_no_mer e_metaphor, accessed January 23, 2016.

118

- "TV retards your child's development" *Consumers Association of Penang.*
  http://www.consumer.org.my/index.php/development/education/34 7-tv-retards-your-childs-development, accessed July 17, 2016.

- Emma Henderson. "Watching lots of TV 'makes you stupid'" *The Independent.* http://www.independent.co.uk/news/science/watching-lots-of-tv-makes-you-stupid-says-american-universities-a6759026.html, December 3, 2015.
- Herbert E. Krugman and Eugene L. Hartley. "Passive Learning From Television" *The Public Opinion Quarterly,* Vol. 34, No. 2. (Oxford University Press, 1970) pp. 184-190.
- Herbert E. Krugman. "Brain Wave Measures of Media Involvement" *How Advertising Works: The Role of Research.* (New York SAGE Publications, 1998) pp. 139–151.
- "Your brain waves change when you watch TV" *I Am Awake.* http://www.iamawake.co/your-brain-waves-change-when-you-watch-tv/, October 11, 2013.
- Kristina Birdsong. "This is Your Child's Brain on TV" *Scientific Learning.* http://www.scilearn.com/blog/how-television-impacts-learning, Mar 22, 2016.
- Douglas Fields. "Watching TV Alters Children's Brain Structure and Lowers IQ". http://rdouglasfields.com/2015/05/watching-tv-alters-childrens-brain-structure-and-lowers-iq/, May 4, 2015.
- Jamil Zaki. "What, Me Care? Young Are Less Empathetic" *Scientific American*. A recent study finds a decline in empathy among young people in the U.S. http://www.scientificamerican.com/article/what-me-care/, December 23, 2010.
- "Children who watch 'excessive' amounts of TV are more likely to have criminal convictions, exhibit aggression and experience negative emotions: study." *New York Daily News*. http://www.nydailynews.com/life-style/health/kids-watch-excessive-tv-criminal-convictions-young-adulthood-study-article-1.1267868, February 19, 2013.
"With every hour in front of the television, kids were more likely to show aggressive behavior or receive a criminal conviction by early adulthood, according to a study published in 'Pediatrics.' The issue isn't necessarily the content of the programming, but the social isolation that comes from so many hours in front of the tube."

- David L. Hill. "Why to Avoid TV Before Age 2" (early brain development). *American Academy of Pediatrics*. http://www.healthychildren.org/English/family-life/Media/Pages/Why-to-Avoid-TV-Before-Age-2.aspx, May 11, 2013. Original Source: Dad to Dad: Parenting Like a Pro (Copyright © American Academy of Pediatrics 2012).
- Alice Park. "Baby Einsteins: Not So Smart After All" *Time*. http://content.time.com/time/health/article/0,8599,1650352,00.html August 06, 2007.
- "Television vs. Reading" *Parent Soup*®, a Trademark of iVillage[sm] Inc. Copyright 1996. http://webshare.northseattle.edu/fam180/topics/tv/tvvsread.htm, accessed May 29, 2014. From Jim Trelease. *The Read-Aloud Handbook*, Penguin Books, 1995.
- "What Children are NOT Doing When Watching TV" *American Academy of Pediatrics*. http://www.healthychildren.org/English/family-life/Media/Pages/What-Children-are-NOT-Doing-When-Watching-TV.aspx, May 11, 2013. Original Source: *Caring for Your School-Age Child: Ages 5 to 12* (Copyright © 2004 American Academy of Pediatrics).
- Marie Winn. "Television and the Brain," "Brain Changes," "Losing the Thread," "The Basic Building Blocks," "A Preference for Watching," "Free Time and Resourcefulness" *Plug-In Drug*. (New York: Viking Penguin, 1977, Revised and Updated Edition, 2002) pp. 67–69, 95–99, 131. From pp. 67–69:
  "'Research conducted during the next two decades removed any doubt about the impact of early brain stimulation on a child's later cognitive development. … they were able to demonstrate that environmental factors can alter neuron pathways during early childhood and long after … among the most important of the environmental factors … are the language and eye contact an infant is exposed to [and] … the number of words an infant hears each day is the single most important predictor of later intelligence, school success and social competence. But there's one catch. The words have to come from an attentive, engaged human being … radio and television do not work."

119

- "What Children are NOT Doing When Watching TV" *American Academy of Pediatrics*.
  http://www.healthychildren.org/English/family-life/Media/Pages/What-Children-are-NOT-Doing-When-Watching-TV.aspx, May 11, 2013.
  Original Source: *Caring for Your School-Age Child: Ages 5 to 12* (Copyright © 2004 American Academy of Pediatrics).
- Marie Winn. "Losing the Thread," "The Basic Building Blocks," "A Preference for Watching," "Free Time and Resourcefulness" *Plug-In Drug*. (New York: Viking Penguin, 1977, Revised and Updated Edition, 2002) pp. 95–99, 131.
- Alice Park. "Baby Einsteins: Not So Smart After All" *Time*.
  http://content.time.com/time/health/article/0,8599,1650352,00.html August 06, 2007.

120

- "Television History - The First 75 Years" *TVhistory.TV*. © 2001-2013. http://www.tvhistory.tv/facts-stats.htm.

121

- "Children who watch 'excessive' amounts of TV are more likely to have criminal convictions, exhibit aggression and experience negative emotions: study" *New York Daily News*.
  http://www.nydailynews.com/life-style/health/kids-watch-excessive-tv-criminal-convictions-young-adulthood-study-article-1.1267868, February 19, 2013.
- Douglas Fields. "Watching TV Alters Children's Brain Structure and Lowers IQ".
  http://rdouglasfields.com/2015/05/watching-tv-alters-childrens-brain-structure-and-lowers-iq/, May 4, 2015.

122

- "Children who watch 'excessive' amounts of TV are more likely to have criminal convictions, exhibit aggression and experience negative emotions: study" *New York Daily News.* http://www.nydailynews.com/life-style/health/kids-watch-excessive-tv-criminal-convictions-young-adulthood-study-article-1.1267868, February 19, 2013.
- Douglas Fields. "Watching TV Alters Children's Brain Structure and Lowers IQ". http://rdouglasfields.com/2015/05/watching-tv-alters-childrens-brain-structure-and-lowers-iq/, May 4, 2015.

123

- Jamil Zaki. "What, Me Care? Young Are Less Empathetic" *Scientific American.* A recent study finds a decline in empathy among young people in the U.S. http://www.scientificamerican.com/article/what-me-care/, December 23, 2010.
- "Children who watch 'excessive' amounts of TV are more likely to have criminal convictions, exhibit aggression and experience negative emotions: study." *New York Daily News.* http://www.nydailynews.com/life-style/health/kids-watch-excessive-tv-criminal-convictions-young-adulthood-study-article-1.1267868, February 19, 2013. "With every hour in front of the television, kids were more likely to show aggressive behavior or receive a criminal conviction by early adulthood, according to a study published in 'Pediatrics.' The issue isn't necessarily the content of the programming, but the social isolation that comes from so many hours in front of the tube."
- "TV retards your child's development" *Consumers Association of Penang.* http://www.consumer.org.my/index.php/development/education/347-tv-retards-your-childs-development, accessed July 17, 2016.

124

- Jamil Zaki. "What, Me Care? Young Are Less Empathetic" *Scientific American*. A recent study finds a decline in empathy among young people in the U.S.
  http://www.scientificamerican.com/article/what-me-care/, December 23, 2010.
- "Children who watch 'excessive' amounts of TV are more likely to have criminal convictions, exhibit aggression and experience negative emotions: study." *New York Daily News*.
  http://www.nydailynews.com/life-style/health/kids-watch-excessive-tv-criminal-convictions-young-adulthood-study-article-1.1267868, February 19, 2013.
  "With every hour in front of the television, kids were more likely to show aggressive behavior or receive a criminal conviction by early adulthood, according to a study published in 'Pediatrics.' The issue isn't necessarily the content of the programming, but the social isolation that comes from so many hours in front of the tube."
- "TV retards your child's development" *Consumers Association of Penang.*
  http://www.consumer.org.my/index.php/development/education/347-tv-retards-your-childs-development, accessed July 17, 2016.

125

- Travis Bradberry. "Eight Habits of Considerate People".
  https://www.linkedin.com/pulse/eight-habits-considerate-people-dr-travis-bradberry, November 8, 2017.

126

- Travis Bradberry. "12 Habits of Genuine People".
  https://www.linkedin.com/pulse/importance-being-genuine-dr-travis-bradberry/, November 15, 2015.

127

- Jamil Zaki. "What, Me Care? Young Are Less Empathetic" *Scientific American*. A recent study finds a decline in empathy among young people in the U.S.
  http://www.scientificamerican.com/article/what-me-care/, December 23, 2010.

- "Children who watch 'excessive' amounts of TV are more likely to have criminal convictions, exhibit aggression and experience negative emotions: study." *New York Daily News*. http://www.nydailynews.com/life-style/health/kids-watch-excessive-tv-criminal-convictions-young-adulthood-study-article-1.1267868, February 19, 2013.
"With every hour in front of the television, kids were more likely to show aggressive behavior or receive a criminal conviction by early adulthood, according to a study published in 'Pediatrics.' The issue isn't necessarily the content of the programming, but the social isolation that comes from so many hours in front of the tube."

128

- Jamil Zaki. "What, Me Care? Young Are Less Empathetic" *Scientific American*. A recent study finds a decline in empathy among young people in the U.S. http://www.scientificamerican.com/article/what-me-care/, December 23, 2010.
- "Children who watch 'excessive' amounts of TV are more likely to have criminal convictions, exhibit aggression and experience negative emotions: study." *New York Daily News*. http://www.nydailynews.com/life-style/health/kids-watch-excessive-tv-criminal-convictions-young-adulthood-study-article-1.1267868, February 19, 2013.
"With every hour in front of the television, kids were more likely to show aggressive behavior or receive a criminal conviction by early adulthood, according to a study published in 'Pediatrics.' The issue isn't necessarily the content of the programming, but the social isolation that comes from so many hours in front of the tube."
- "TV retards your child's development" *Consumers Association of Penang*. http://www.consumer.org.my/index.php/development/education/34 7-tv-retards-your-childs-development, accessed July 17, 2016.

129

- Herbert E. Krugman and Eugene L. Hartley. "Passive Learning From Television" *The Public Opinion Quarterly,* Vol. 34, No. 2. (Oxford University Press, 1970) pp. 184-190.

- Herbert E. Krugman. "Brain Wave Measures of Media Involvement" *How Advertising Works: The Role of Research.* (New York SAGE Publications, 1998) pp. 139–151.
- "Your brain waves change when you watch TV" *I Am Awake.* http://www.iamawake.co/your-brain-waves-change-when-you-watch-tv/, October 11, 2013.

130

- Claudine Ryan. "Why is watching TV so bad for you?" *ABC Health & Wellbeing.* http://www.abc.net.au/health/thepulse/stories/2014/07/24/4043618.htm, July 24, 2014.

131

- Amanda Gardner. "TV watching raises risk of health problems, dying young" *CNN.* http://www.cnn.com/2011/HEALTH/06/14/tv.watching.unhealthy/, June 14, 2011.
  - "For every two hours Americans spend watching TV each day, there are 176 new cases of diabetes, 38 additional deaths from heart disease, and 104 additional deaths due to any cause per 100,000 people per year"—That's 2 hours/day per 100,000 people. That means given the US population of 324,000,000, and the fact that average US TV viewing is 4 hours per day—TV viewing causes a total of 1,140,480 new cases of diabetes, 246,240 additional deaths from heart disease, and 673,920 additional deaths, every year.

132

- Amanda Gardner. "TV watching raises risk of health problems, dying young" *CNN.* http://www.cnn.com/2011/HEALTH/06/14/tv.watching.unhealthy/, June 14, 2011.

- "For every two hours Americans spend watching TV each day, there are 176 new cases of diabetes, 38 additional deaths from heart disease, and 104 additional deaths due to any cause per 100,000 people per year"—That's 2 hours/day per 100,000 people. That means given the US population of 324,000,000, and the fact that average US TV viewing is 4 hours per day—TV viewing causes a total of 1,140,480 new cases of diabetes, 246,240 additional deaths from heart disease, and 673,920 additional deaths, every year.

133

- Herbert E. Krugman and Eugene L. Hartley. "Passive Learning From Television" *The Public Opinion Quarterly,* Vol. 34, No. 2. (Oxford University Press, 1970) pp. 184-190.
- Herbert E. Krugman. "Brain Wave Measures of Media Involvement" *How Advertising Works: The Role of Research.* (New York SAGE Publications, 1998) pp. 139–151.
- "Your brain waves change when you watch TV" *I Am Awake.* http://www.iamawake.co/your-brain-waves-change-when-you-watch-tv/, October 11, 2013.
- Allan Stromfeldt Christensen. "Lemminged: to be herded off the peak oil cliff by filmmakers" *TransitionVoice.com.* http://transitionvoice.com/2014/11/lemminged-to-be-herded-off-the-peak-oil-cliff-by-filmmakers/, November 11, 2014.
- "Television: Opiate of the Masses" *FamilyResource.com.* http://www.familyresource.com/lifestyles/mental-environment/television-opiate-of-the-masses, accessed May 29, 2014.
- Douglas Fields. "Watching TV Alters Children's Brain Structure and Lowers IQ". http://rdouglasfields.com/2015/05/watching-tv-alters-childrens-brain-structure-and-lowers-iq/, May 4, 2015.
- Kristina Birdsong. "This is Your Child's Brain on TV" *Scientific Learning.* http://www.scilearn.com/blog/how-television-impacts-learning, Mar 22, 2016.

134

- Tom Nichols. *The Death of Expertise.* p. 143. New York: Oxford University Press, 2017.

135

- Robert Kubey and Mihaly Csikszentmihalyi. "Television Addiction is no mere metaphor" *Scientific American.* http://www.academia.edu/5065840/Television_Addiction_is_no_mere_metaphor, accessed January 23, 2016.

136

- Herbert E. Krugman and Eugene L. Hartley. "Passive Learning From Television" *The Public Opinion Quarterly,* Vol. 34, No. 2. (Oxford University Press, 1970) pp. 184-190.
- Herbert E. Krugman. "Brain Wave Measures of Media Involvement" *How Advertising Works: The Role of Research.* (New York SAGE Publications, 1998) pp. 139–151.
- "Your brain waves change when you watch TV" *I Am Awake.* http://www.iamawake.co/your-brain-waves-change-when-you-watch-tv/, October 11, 2013.
- "Television: Opiate of the Masses" *FamilyResource.com.* http://www.familyresource.com/lifestyles/mental-environment/television-opiate-of-the-masses, accessed May 29, 2014.
- Douglas Fields. "Watching TV Alters Children's Brain Structure and Lowers IQ". http://rdouglasfields.com/2015/05/watching-tv-alters-childrens-brain-structure-and-lowers-iq/, May 4, 2015.
- Kristina Birdsong. "This is Your Child's Brain on TV" *Scientific Learning.* http://www.scilearn.com/blog/how-television-impacts-learning, Mar 22, 2016.

137

- David Hinckley. "Average American watches 5 hours of TV per day, report shows Time spent watching live TV increases steadily as we get older, according to a new report from Nielsen" *New York Daily News.* http://nydn.us/1fHRJee, Wednesday, March 5, 2014, 5:27 p.m.

- Per Nielsen, here's the average weekly usage for ascending age groups. Ages:
  - 2–11: 24 hours, 16 minutes. (round down to 24 hours, 15 minutes, or 24.25 x 10 years counting ages 2 and 11 = 12,610)
  - 12–17: 20 hours, 41 minutes. (round down to 20 hours, 30 minutes, or 20.5 hours x 6 years counting ages 12 and 17 = 6,396)
  - 18–24: 22 hours, 27 minutes. (round down to 22 hours, 20 minutes, or 20.33 hours x 6 years counting age 18 to end of age 23 = 6,343)
- By age 24, the average American has watched 25,349 hours of TV (does not include PC/Internet video time). Here is the breakdown continuing older age groups, showing people watch more and more as they get older. Ages:
  - 25–34: 27 hours, 36 minutes.
  - 35–49: 33 hours, 40 minutes.
  - 50–64: 43 hours, 56 minutes.
  - 65–plus: 50 hours, 34 minutes.
- Victor C. Strasburger, MD, FAAP, and Marjorie J. Hogan, MD, FAAP. "Children, Adolescents, and the Media" *American Academy of Pediatrics.* http://pediatrics.aappublications.org/content/132/5/958.full, May 11, 2013.

138

- "TV retards your child's development" *Consumers Association of Penang.* http://www.consumer.org.my/index.php/development/education/347-tv-retards-your-childs-development, accessed July 17, 2016.
- Emma Henderson. "Watching lots of TV 'makes you stupid'" *The Independent.* http://www.independent.co.uk/news/science/watching-lots-of-tv-makes-you-stupid-says-american-universities-a6759026.html, December 3, 2015.
- Herbert E. Krugman and Eugene L. Hartley. "Passive Learning From Television" *The Public Opinion Quarterly,* Vol. 34, No. 2. (Oxford University Press, 1970) pp. 184-190.

- Herbert E. Krugman. "Brain Wave Measures of Media Involvement" *How Advertising Works: The Role of Research.* (New York SAGE Publications, 1998) pp. 139–151.
- "Your brain waves change when you watch TV" *I Am Awake.* http://www.iamawake.co/your-brain-waves-change-when-you-watch-tv/, October 11, 2013.
- Kristina Birdsong. "This is Your Child's Brain on TV" *Scientific Learning.* http://www.scilearn.com/blog/how-television-impacts-learning, Mar 22, 2016.
- Douglas Fields. "Watching TV Alters Children's Brain Structure and Lowers IQ". http://rdouglasfields.com/2015/05/watching-tv-alters-childrens-brain-structure-and-lowers-iq/, May 4, 2015.
- Jamil Zaki. "What, Me Care? Young Are Less Empathetic" *Scientific American.* A recent study finds a decline in empathy among young people in the U.S. http://www.scientificamerican.com/article/what-me-care/, December 23, 2010.
- "Children who watch 'excessive' amounts of TV are more likely to have criminal convictions, exhibit aggression and experience negative emotions: study." *New York Daily News.* http://www.nydailynews.com/life-style/health/kids-watch-excessive-tv-criminal-convictions-young-adulthood-study-article-1.1267868, February 19, 2013.
  "With every hour in front of the television, kids were more likely to show aggressive behavior or receive a criminal conviction by early adulthood, according to a study published in 'Pediatrics.' The issue isn't necessarily the content of the programming, but the social isolation that comes from so many hours in front of the tube."
- David L. Hill. "Why to Avoid TV Before Age 2" (early brain development). *American Academy of Pediatrics.* http://www.healthychildren.org/English/family-life/Media/Pages/Why-to-Avoid-TV-Before-Age-2.aspx, May 11, 2013. Original Source: Dad to Dad: Parenting Like a Pro (Copyright © American Academy of Pediatrics 2012).

- Alice Park. "Baby Einsteins: Not So Smart After All" *Time*. http://content.time.com/time/health/article/0,8599,1650352,00.html August 06, 2007.
- "Television vs. Reading" *Parent Soup*®, a Trademark of iVillage℠ Inc. Copyright 1996. http://webshare.northseattle.edu/fam180/topics/tv/tvvsread.htm, accessed May 29, 2014.
  From Jim Trelease. *The Read-Aloud Handbook*, Penguin Books, 1995.
- "What Children are NOT Doing When Watching TV" *American Academy of Pediatrics*. http://www.healthychildren.org/English/family-life/Media/Pages/What-Children-are-NOT-Doing-When-Watching-TV.aspx, May 11, 2013.
  Original Source: *Caring for Your School-Age Child: Ages 5 to 12* (Copyright © 2004 American Academy of Pediatrics).
- Tina D. Hoang, MSPH; Jared Reis, PhD; Na Zhu, MD, MPH; David R. Jacobs Jr, PhD; Lenore J. Launer, PhD; Rachel A. Whitmer, PhD; Stephen Sidney, MD; Kristine Yaffe, MD.
  "Effect of Early Adult Patterns of Physical Activity and Television Viewing on Midlife Cognitive Function" *JAMA Psychiatry* (The Journal of the American Medical Association). http://archpsyc.jamanetwork.com/article.aspx?articleid=2471270, January 2016, Vol 73, No. 1.
- Marie Winn. "Television and the Brain," "Brain Changes," "Losing the Thread," "The Basic Building Blocks," "A Preference for Watching," "Free Time and Resourcefulness" *Plug-In Drug.* (New York: Viking Penguin, 1977, Revised and Updated Edition, 2002) pp. 67–69, 95–99, 131.

139

- Tom Nichols. *The Death of Expertise.* p. 99. New York: Oxford University Press, 2017.

140

- Jeff Haden. *The Motivation Myth.* p. 16. New York: Penguin, 2018.

141

- Jeff Haden. *The Motivation Myth.* p. 15. New York: Penguin, 2018.

142

- Ana Tintocalis. "San Francisco Middle Schools No Longer Teaching 'Algebra 1'" *The California Report*, KQED News. http://ww2.kqed.org/news/2015/07/22/san-francisco-middle-schools-no-longer-teaching-algebra-1, July 22, 2015.

143

- Caroline McCarthy. "Hulu: We're evil, and proud of it" *CNet*. https://www.cnet.com/news/hulu-were-evil-and-proud-of-it/, February 2, 2009.
  The example video: https://youtu.be/Ek8T4F1ZHG8.

144

- Catherine Rampell. "The rise of the 'gentleman's A' and the GPA arms race" *The Washington Post*. https://www.washingtonpost.com/opinions/the-rise-of-the-gentlemans-a-and-the-gpa-arms-race/2016/03/28/05c9e966-f522-11e5-9804-537defcc3cf6_story.html, March 28, 2016.

145

- Emma Henderson. "Watching lots of TV 'makes you stupid'" *The Independent*. http://www.independent.co.uk/news/science/watching-lots-of-tv-makes-you-stupid-says-american-universities-a6759026.html, December 3, 2015.
- Tina D. Hoang, MSPH; Jared Reis, PhD; Na Zhu, MD, MPH; David R. Jacobs Jr, PhD; Lenore J. Launer, PhD; Rachel A. Whitmer, PhD; Stephen Sidney, MD; Kristine Yaffe, MD. "Effect of Early Adult Patterns of Physical Activity and Television Viewing on Midlife Cognitive Function" *JAMA Psychiatry* (The Journal of the American Medical Association). http://archpsyc.jamanetwork.com/article.aspx?articleid=2471270, January 2016, Vol 73, No. 1.

146

- Catherine Rampell. "The rise of the 'gentleman's A' and the GPA arms race" *The Washington Post.*
  https://www.washingtonpost.com/opinions/the-rise-of-the-gentlemans-a-and-the-gpa-arms-race/2016/03/28/05c9e966-f522-11e5-9804-537defcc3cf6_story.html, March 28, 2016.

147

- Ray Williams. "Anti-Intellectualism and the 'Dumbing Down' of America" *Psychology Today.*
  https://www.psychologytoday.com/blog/wired-success/201407/anti-intellectualism-and-the-dumbing-down-america. July 7, 2014.

148

- Educational Testing Service (ETS). "America's Skills Challenge: Millennials and the Future" *The ETS Center for Research on Human Capital and Education.* Princeton, NJ: January 2015.
  https://www.ets.org/s/research/30079/asc-millennials-and-the-future.pdf.
  Note: The Educational Testing Service (ETS) is the academic organization that administers the SAT tests to high school students bound for college.

149

- Kevin Carey. "Americans Think We Have the World's Best Colleges. We Don't." *The New York Times.*
  https://www.nytimes.com/2014/06/29/upshot/americans-think-we-have-the-worlds-best-colleges-we-dont.html, June 28, 2014.

150

- Tom Nichols. *The Death of Expertise.* p. 93. New York: Oxford University Press, 2017.

151

- Tom Nichols. *The Death of Expertise.* p. 93. New York: Oxford University Press, 2017.

152

- Catherine Rampell. "The rise of the 'gentleman's A' and the GPA arms race" *The Washington Post.* https://www.washingtonpost.com/opinions/the-rise-of-the-gentlemans-a-and-the-gpa-arms-race/2016/03/28/05c9e966-f522-11e5-9804-537defcc3cf6_story.html, March 28, 2016.

153

- Tom Nichols. *The Death of Expertise.* pp. 74–75. New York: Oxford University Press, 2017.

154

- Jeremy Warner. "Harsh truths about the decline of Britain" *The Telegraph.* http://www.telegraph.co.uk/finance/economics/10417838/Harsh-truths-about-the-decline-of-Britain.html, October 31, 2013.

155

- Tom Nichols. *The Death of Expertise.* pp. 72–76. New York: Oxford University Press, 2017.

156

- Tom Nichols. *The Death of Expertise.* p. 94. New York: Oxford University Press, 2017.

157

- Tom Nichols. *The Death of Expertise.* p. 71. New York: Oxford University Press, 2017.

158

- Tom Nichols. *The Death of Expertise.* p. 72. New York: Oxford University Press, 2017.

159

- Scott Jaschik. "Let the Right Ones In" *Slate.com.* http://www.slate.com/articles/life/inside_higher_ed/2014/10/college_admissions_rose_hulman_institute_of_technology_uses_locus_of_control.html, October 30, 2014.

186

160

- Rebecca Schuman. "Welcome to 13th Grade!" *Slate.com*. http://www.slate.com/articles/life/education/2014/10/high_schools_ offer_a_fifth_year_of_high_school_13th_grade_is_a_great_idea.html October 22, 2014.

161

- Rebecca Schuman. "Welcome to 13th Grade!" *Slate.com*. http://www.slate.com/articles/life/education/2014/10/high_schools_ offer_a_fifth_year_of_high_school_13th_grade_is_a_great_idea.html October 22, 2014.

162

- Amy Joyce. "How helicopter parents are ruining college students" *The Washington Post*. http://www.washingtonpost.com/news/parenting/wp/2014/09/02/h ow-helicopter-parents-are-ruining-college-students/, September 2, 2014.

163

- Marie Winn. "Waiting on Children" *Plug-In Drug.* (New York: Viking Penguin, 1977, Revised and Updated Edition, 2002) p. 146.

164

- Sharon Jayson. "Generation Y's goal? Wealth and fame" *USA Today*. http://usatoday30.usatoday.com/news/nation/2007-01-09-gen-y-cover_x.htm, Posted January 9,2007, Updated January 10, 2007.

165

- Amy Joyce. "How helicopter parents are ruining college students" The Washington Post. http://www.washingtonpost.com/news/parenting/wp/2014/09/02/h ow-helicopter-parents-are-ruining-college-students/, September 2, 2014.

166

- "Television Addiction" *All About Life Challenges*. http://www.allaboutlifechallenges.org/television-addiction.htm, accessed September 21, 2014.
- "Television: Opiate of the Masses" *FamilyResource.com*. http://www.familyresource.com/lifestyles/mental-environment/television-opiate-of-the-masses, accessed May 29, 2014.

167

- Celestine Chua. "Top 10 Reasons You Should Stop Watching TV" *Personal Excellence: Be Your Best Self, Live Your Best Life.* http://personalexcellence.co/blog/top-10-reasons-you-should-stop-watching-tv/, May 2, 2010.

168

- Jeff Haden. *The Motivation Myth.* p. 168. New York: Penguin, 2018.

169

- Travis Bradberry and Jean Greaves. *Emotional Intelligence 2.0.* p. 69. San Diego, California: TalentSmart, 2009.

170

- Travis Bradberry and Jean Greaves. *Emotional Intelligence 2.0.* p. 147. San Diego, California: TalentSmart, 2009.

171

- Matt Richtel. "The Myth of Multitasking" *Attached to Technology and Paying a Price*, p. 2. *NYTimes.com*. http://www.nytimes.com/2010/06/07/technology/07brain.html, June 6, 2010.
- Johanna Rothman. "Why Multitasking Doesn't Work" *Pragmatic Manager*. http://www.jrothman.com/2011/01/why-multitasking-doesnt-work/, January 1, 2011.
- Porter Anderson. "Study: Multitasking is counterproductive" *CNN*. http://www.cnn.com/2001/CAREER/trends/08/05/multitasking.study/index.html, December 6, 2001.

172

- Travis Bradberry. "9 Surprising Things Ultra Productive People Do Every Day" https://www.linkedin.com/pulse/surprising-things-ultra-productive-people-do-every-day-bradberry/, November 7, 2016.

173

- Joseph Stromberg. "Why you should take notes by hand — not on a laptop". *Vox: Science & Health*. http://www.vox.com/2014/6/4/5776804/note-taking-by-hand-versus-laptop, March 31, 2015.

174

- Ceridwen Dovey. "Can Reading Make You Happier?" *The New Yorker*. http://www.newyorker.com/culture/cultural-comment/can-reading-make-you-happier, June 9, 2015.

175

- Thu-Huong Ha. "New research links reading books with longer life" *Quartz*. http://qz.com/754109/new-research-links-reading-books-with-longer-life/, August 10, 2016.

176

- Amanda Gardner. "TV watching raises risk of health problems, dying young" *CNN*. http://www.cnn.com/2011/HEALTH/06/14/tv.watching.unhealthy/, June 14, 2011.
  - "For every two hours Americans spend watching TV each day, there are 176 new cases of diabetes, 38 additional deaths from heart disease, and 104 additional deaths due to any cause per 100,000 people per year"—That's 2 hours/day per 100,000 people. That means given the US population of 324,000,000, and the fact that average US TV viewing is 4 hours per day—TV viewing causes a total of 1,140,480 new cases of diabetes, 246,240 additional deaths from heart disease, and 673,920 additional deaths, every year.

177

- "HOME-SCHOOLING: Outstanding results on national tests" *The Washington Times.* http://www.washingtontimes.com/news/2009/aug/30/home-schooling-outstanding-results-national-tests/, August 30, 2009.

178

- EJ Fox and Mike Spies. "Who Was America's Most Well-Spoken President?" *Vocativ.* http://www.vocativ.com/interactive/usa/us-politics/presidential-readability/, October 10, 2014.

179

- Stephen Knott, ed. "Life Before the Presidency" *American President: George Washington (1732–1799), Essays on George Washington and His Administration.* Miller Center, University of Virginia. http://millercenter.org/president/washington/essays/biography/2, accessed November 19, 2014.

180

- EJ Fox and Mike Spies. "Who Was America's Most Well-Spoken President?" *Vocativ.* http://www.vocativ.com/interactive/usa/us-politics/presidential-readability/, October 10, 2014.

181

- Stephen Knott, ed. "Life Before the Presidency" *American President: George Washington (1732–1799), Essays on George Washington and His Administration.* Miller Center, University of Virginia. http://millercenter.org/president/washington/essays/biography/2, accessed November 19, 2014.
- EJ Fox and Mike Spies. "Who Was America's Most Well-Spoken President?" *Vocativ.* http://www.vocativ.com/interactive/usa/us-politics/presidential-readability/, October 10, 2014.

182

- Tom Nichols. *The Death of Expertise.* p. 132. New York: Oxford University Press, 2017.

183

- Shahram Heshmat. "What Is Confirmation Bias?" *Psychology Today.* https://www.psychologytoday.com/blog/science-choice/201504/what-is-confirmation-bias, April 23, 2015.

184

- Tom Nichols. *The Death of Expertise.* pp. 140, 155. New York: Oxford University Press, 2017.

185

- Jeff Grabmeier. "Both liberals, conservatives can have science bias: Study finds different topics bedevil the left and right" *The Ohio State University.* https://news.osu.edu/news/2015/02/09/both-liberals-conservatives-can-have-science-bias/, February 09, 2015.
- Chris Mooney. "Liberals deny science, too" *The Washington Post.* https://www.washingtonpost.com/news/wonk/wp/2014/10/28/liberals-deny-science-too/, October 28, 2014.
- Tom Nichols. *The Death of Expertise.* p. 69. New York: Oxford University Press, 2017.

186

- Melissa Dahl. "How Neuroscientists Explain the Mind-Clearing Magic of Running" Science of Us, *New York Magazine.* http://nymag.com/scienceofus/2016/04/how-neuroscientists-explain-the-mind-clearing-magic-of-running.html, April 21, 2016.

187

- University of Tsukuba. "Active body, active mind: The secret to a younger brain may lie in exercising your body" *ScienceDaily.* http://www.sciencedaily.com/releases/2015/10/151023084456.htm, October 23, 2015.

188

- Travis Bradberry and Jean Greaves. *Emotional Intelligence 2.0.* p. 132. San Diego, California: TalentSmart, 2009.

189

- "Want a younger brain? Stay in school — and take the stairs" *Science Daily.* https://www.sciencedaily.com/releases/2016/03/160309125520.htm March 9, 2016.

190

- Celestine Chua. "Top 10 Reasons You Should Stop Watching TV" *Personal Excellence: Be Your Best Self, Live Your Best Life.* http://personalexcellence.co/blog/top-10-reasons-you-should-stop-watching-tv/, May 2, 2010.

191

- "Children who watch 'excessive' amounts of TV are more likely to have criminal convictions, exhibit aggression and experience negative emotions: study." *New York Daily News.* http://www.nydailynews.com/life-style/health/kids-watch-excessive-tv-criminal-convictions-young-adulthood-study-article-1.1267868, February 19, 2013. "With every hour in front of the television, kids were more likely to show aggressive behavior or receive a criminal conviction by early adulthood, according to a study published in 'Pediatrics.' The issue isn't necessarily the content of the programming, but the social isolation that comes from so many hours in front of the tube."

192

- Travis Bradberry. "13 Things Mentally Strong People Won't Do". https://www.linkedin.com/pulse/13-things-mentally-strong-people-wont-do-dr-travis-bradberry/, September 11, 2017.

193

- Travis Bradberry and Jean Greaves. *Emotional Intelligence 2.0.* p. 196. San Diego, California: TalentSmart, 2009.

194

- Travis Bradberry and Jean Greaves. *Emotional Intelligence 2.0.* pp. 52, 53. San Diego, California: TalentSmart, 2009.

195

- Travis Bradberry and Jean Greaves. *Emotional Intelligence 2.0.* p. 237. San Diego, California: TalentSmart, 2009.

196

- Travis Bradberry. "Eight Habits of Considerate People". https://www.linkedin.com/pulse/eight-habits-considerate-people-dr-travis-bradberry, November 8, 2017.

197

- Travis Bradberry and Jean Greaves. *Emotional Intelligence 2.0.* pp. 244, 245. San Diego, California: TalentSmart, 2009.

198

- Travis Bradberry. "13 Things Mentally Strong People Won't Do". https://www.linkedin.com/pulse/13-things-mentally-strong-people-wont-do-dr-travis-bradberry/, September 11, 2017.

199

- Travis Bradberry and Jean Greaves. *Emotional Intelligence 2.0.* p. 245. San Diego, California: TalentSmart, 2009.

200

- Travis Bradberry and Jean Greaves. *Emotional Intelligence 2.0.* p. 75. San Diego, California: TalentSmart, 2009.

201

- Travis Bradberry. "These are the habits that mentally strong people rely on" *World Economic Forum.* https://www.weforum.org/agenda/2016/10/habits-to-help-you-develop-mental-strength, October 26, 2016.

202

- Travis Bradberry. "9 Habits of Profoundly Influential People". https://www.linkedin.com/pulse/critical-habits-profoundly-influential-people-dr-travis-bradberry/, July 20, 2015.

203

- Travis Bradberry. "12 Habits of Genuine People". https://www.linkedin.com/pulse/importance-being-genuine-dr-travis-bradberry/, November 15, 2015.

204

- Leslie Becker-Phelps. "Don't Just React: Choose Your Response" *Psychology Today.* https://www.psychologytoday.com/blog/making-change/201307/dont-just-react-choose-your-response, July 23, 2013.

205

- Leslie Becker-Phelps. "Don't Just React: Choose Your Response" *Psychology Today.* https://www.psychologytoday.com/blog/making-change/201307/dont-just-react-choose-your-response, July 23, 2013.

206

- Jamil Zaki. "What, Me Care? Young Are Less Empathetic" *Scientific American*. A recent study finds a decline in empathy among young people in the U.S. http://www.scientificamerican.com/article/what-me-care/, December 23, 2010.

- "Children who watch 'excessive' amounts of TV are more likely to have criminal convictions, exhibit aggression and experience negative emotions: study." *New York Daily News*. http://www.nydailynews.com/life-style/health/kids-watch-excessive-tv-criminal-convictions-young-adulthood-study-article-1.1267868, February 19, 2013.
"With every hour in front of the television, kids were more likely to show aggressive behavior or receive a criminal conviction by early adulthood, according to a study published in 'Pediatrics.' The issue isn't necessarily the content of the programming, but the social isolation that comes from so many hours in front of the tube."
- "TV retards your child's development" *Consumers Association of Penang*. http://www.consumer.org.my/index.php/development/education/347-tv-retards-your-childs-development, accessed July 17, 2016.

207

- "Children who watch 'excessive' amounts of TV are more likely to have criminal convictions, exhibit aggression and experience negative emotions: study" *New York Daily News*. http://www.nydailynews.com/life-style/health/kids-watch-excessive-tv-criminal-convictions-young-adulthood-study-article-1.1267868, February 19, 2013.
- Douglas Fields. "Watching TV Alters Children's Brain Structure and Lowers IQ". http://rdouglasfields.com/2015/05/watching-tv-alters-childrens-brain-structure-and-lowers-iq/, May 4, 2015.

208

- Hugh Wilson. "Are men becoming more feminine?" *MSN.com*. http://him.uk.msn.com/in-the-know/are-men-becoming-more-feminine-women-male-female-gender-gap, July 19, 2013.
- "Gender Switch: When Did Men Become So Feminine?" *Urban Belle*. http://urbanbellemag.com/2010/10/gender-switch-when-did-men-become-so-feminine.html, October 18, 2010

- "Since 2010, there has been a rise of men's rights movements in regions around Europe and the United States. These movements seek to advocate for the rights of fathers, and support the changing masculine roles in relationships. According to research studies, the women have outnumbered men in high paying jobs; it is evident that in the modern family set ups a large number of men are taking up the feminine roles."
  "Masculine And Feminine Roles In Relationships Sociology Essay" *Essays, UK.*
  http://www.ukessays.com/essays/sociology/masculine-and-feminine-roles-in-relationships-sociology-essay.php?cref=1, November 2013.

209

- Christopher Ingraham. "Today's men are not nearly as strong as their dads were, researchers say" *Washington Post.*
  https://www.washingtonpost.com/news/wonk/wp/2016/08/15/todays-men-are-nowhere-near-as-strong-as-their-dads-were-researchers-say/, August 15, 2016.

210

- "Masculine And Feminine Roles In Relationships Sociology Essay" *Essays, UK.*
  http://www.ukessays.com/essays/sociology/masculine-and-feminine-roles-in-relationships-sociology-essay.php?cref=1, November 2013. "Since 2010 ... it is evident that in the modern family set ups a large number of men are taking up the feminine roles."
- Hugh Wilson. "Are men becoming more feminine?" *MSN.com.*
  http://him.uk.msn.com/in-the-know/are-men-becoming-more-feminine-women-male-female-gender-gap, July 19, 2013.
- "Gender Switch: When Did Men Become So Feminine?" *Urban Belle.*
  http://urbanbellemag.com/2010/10/gender-switch-when-did-men-become-so-feminine.html, October 18, 2010

211

- "Physical Fighting by Youth" *Child Trends Databank.*
  https://www.childtrends.org/indicators/physical-fighting-by-youth/, Accessed December 23, 2017.

- "Gender Switch: When Did Men Become So Feminine?" *Urban Belle*. http://urbanbellemag.com/2010/10/gender-switch-when-did-men-become-so-feminine.html, October 18, 2010
- Hugh Wilson. "Are men becoming more feminine?" *MSN.com*. http://him.uk.msn.com/in-the-know/are-men-becoming-more-feminine-women-male-female-gender-gap, July 19, 2013.

212

- "Physical Fighting by Youth" *Child Trends Databank*. https://www.childtrends.org/indicators/physical-fighting-by-youth/, Accessed December 23, 2017.

213

- Sergio M. Pellis and Vivien C. Pellis. "Rough-and-Tumble Play: Training and Using the Social Brain" *The Oxford Handbook of the Development of Play* (December 2010).
  Online Reference:
  http://www.oxfordhandbooks.com/view/10.1093/oxfordhb/9780195393002.001.0001/oxfordhb-9780195393002-e-019, September 2012.
- Eileen Kennedy-Moore. "Do Boys Need Rough and Tumble Play?" *Psychology Today*. https://www.psychologytoday.com/blog/growing-friendships/201506/do-boys-need-rough-and-tumble-play, June 30, 2015.

214

- Eileen Kennedy-Moore. "Do Boys Need Rough and Tumble Play?" *Psychology Today*. https://www.psychologytoday.com/blog/growing-friendships/201506/do-boys-need-rough-and-tumble-play, June 30, 2015.
- Peter K. Smith. "Chapter 6: Physical Activity Play: Exercise Play and Rough-and-Tumble" *Children and Play* (April 2009).
  Online Reference:
  http://onlinelibrary.wiley.com/doi/10.1002/9781444311006.ch6/summary, April 24, 2009.

215

- "ISU study finds TV viewing, video game play contribute to kids' attention problems" *Iowa State University*. http://www.news.iastate.edu/news/2010/jul/TVVGattention, July 4, 2010.

216

- Eileen Kennedy-Moore. "Do Boys Need Rough and Tumble Play?" *Psychology Today*. https://www.psychologytoday.com/blog/growing-friendships/201506/do-boys-need-rough-and-tumble-play, June 30, 2015.
- Jaak Panksepp. "Can PLAY diminish ADHD and facilitate the construction of the social brain?" *Journal of the Canadian Academy of Child and Adolescent Psychiatry* (16, 57-66), 2007.

217

- "Children who watch 'excessive' amounts of TV are more likely to have criminal convictions, exhibit aggression and experience negative emotions: study." *New York Daily News*. http://www.nydailynews.com/life-style/health/kids-watch-excessive-tv-criminal-convictions-young-adulthood-study-article-1.1267868, February 19, 2013.
  "With every hour in front of the television, kids were more likely to show aggressive behavior or receive a criminal conviction by early adulthood, according to a study published in 'Pediatrics.' The issue isn't necessarily the content of the programming, but the social isolation that comes from so many hours in front of the tube."

218

- "Children who watch 'excessive' amounts of TV are more likely to have criminal convictions, exhibit aggression and experience negative emotions: study." *New York Daily News.* http://www.nydailynews.com/life-style/health/kids-watch-excessive-tv-criminal-convictions-young-adulthood-study-article-1.1267868, February 19, 2013.
"With every hour in front of the television, kids were more likely to show aggressive behavior or receive a criminal conviction by early adulthood, according to a study published in 'Pediatrics.' The issue isn't necessarily the content of the programming, but the social isolation that comes from so many hours in front of the tube."

219

- Travis Bradberry. "10 Things Mentally Strong People Won't Do". https://www.forbes.com/sites/travisbradberry/2016/09/20/10-things-mentally-strong-people-wont-do/, September 20, 2016.

220

- Jeff Haden. *The Motivation Myth.* p. 17. New York: Penguin, 2018.

221

- Travis Bradberry and Jean Greaves. *Emotional Intelligence 2.0.* pp. 119. San Diego, California: TalentSmart, 2009.

222

- Travis Bradberry. "13 Things Mentally Strong People Won't Do". https://www.linkedin.com/pulse/13-things-mentally-strong-people-wont-do-dr-travis-bradberry/, September 11, 2017.

223

- Jim Taylor. "Parenting: The Sad Misuse of Self-esteem" *Psychology Today.* https://www.psychologytoday.com/blog/the-power-prime/201002/parenting-the-sad-misuse-self-esteem, February 22, 2010.

224

- Travis Bradberry. "These are the habits that mentally strong people rely on" *World Economic Forum.* https://www.weforum.org/agenda/2016/10/habits-to-help-you-develop-mental-strength, October 26, 2016.

225

- Jeff Haden. *The Motivation Myth.* pp. 28–29. New York: Penguin, 2018.

226

- Peter M. Gollwitzer et al., "When Intentions Go Public: Does Social Reality Widen the Intention-Behavior Gap?" *Psychological Science* 20, no. 5 (May 1, 2009): 612. http://journals.sagepub.com/doi/abs/10.1111/j.1467-9280.2009.02336.x, May 1, 2009.
- Jeff Haden. *The Motivation Myth.* p. 28. New York: Penguin, 2018.

227

- Peter M. Gollwitzer et al., "When Intentions Go Public: Does Social Reality Widen the Intention-Behavior Gap?" *Psychological Science* 20, no. 5 (May 1, 2009): 612. http://journals.sagepub.com/doi/abs/10.1111/j.1467-9280.2009.02336.x, May 1, 2009.

228

- Travis Bradberry and Jean Greaves. *Emotional Intelligence 2.0.* p. 68. San Diego, California: TalentSmart, 2009.

229

- Jim Taylor. "Parenting: The Sad Misuse of Self-esteem" *Psychology Today.* https://www.psychologytoday.com/blog/the-power-prime/201002/parenting-the-sad-misuse-self-esteem, February 22, 2010.

230

- Travis Bradberry. "13 Things Mentally Strong People Won't Do". https://www.linkedin.com/pulse/13-things-mentally-strong-people-wont-do-dr-travis-bradberry/, September 11, 2017.

231

- Travis Bradberry. "12 Habits of Genuine People". https://www.linkedin.com/pulse/importance-being-genuine-dr-travis-bradberry/, November 15, 2015.

232

- Travis Bradberry. "13 Things Mentally Strong People Won't Do". https://www.linkedin.com/pulse/13-things-mentally-strong-people-wont-do-dr-travis-bradberry/, September 11, 2017.

233

- William Frierson. "Dream vs. Reality: What Happens After Graduation" *College Recruiter*. https://www.collegerecruiter.com/blog/2015/07/14/dream-vs-reality-what-happens-after-graduation/, July 14, 2015.

234

- Carrie Courogen. "9 Harsh Realities About Graduating College That I Wish Someone Had Warned Me About" *Bustle*. https://www.bustle.com/articles/80461-9-harsh-realities-about-graduating-college-that-i-wish-someone-had-warned-me-about, May 4, 2015.

235

- Travis Bradberry. "13 Things Mentally Strong People Won't Do". https://www.linkedin.com/pulse/13-things-mentally-strong-people-wont-do-dr-travis-bradberry/, September 11, 2017.

236

- Jeff Haden. *The Motivation Myth.* p. 236. New York: Penguin, 2018.

237

- Jeff Haden. *The Motivation Myth.* p. 180. New York: Penguin, 2018.

238

- Jeff Haden. *The Motivation Myth.* p. 9. New York: Penguin, 2018.

239

- Travis Bradberry. "11 Things Ultra-Productive People Do Differently" *Forbes.* https://www.forbes.com/sites/travisbradberry/2015/05/13/11-things-ultra-productive-people-do-differently/, May 13, 2015.

240

- Travis Bradberry. "These are the habits that mentally strong people rely on" *World Economic Forum.* https://www.weforum.org/agenda/2016/10/habits-to-help-you-develop-mental-strength, October 26, 2016.

241

- Jeff Haden. *The Motivation Myth.* p. 132–135, 140. New York: Penguin, 2018.

242

- Travis Bradberry. "These are the habits that mentally strong people rely on" *World Economic Forum.* https://www.weforum.org/agenda/2016/10/habits-to-help-you-develop-mental-strength, October 26, 2016.

243

- Travis Bradberry. "These are the habits that mentally strong people rely on" *World Economic Forum.* https://www.weforum.org/agenda/2016/10/habits-to-help-you-develop-mental-strength, October 26, 2016.

244

- Travis Bradberry. "These are the habits that mentally strong people rely on" *World Economic Forum.* https://www.weforum.org/agenda/2016/10/habits-to-help-you-develop-mental-strength, October 26, 2016.

245

- Travis Bradberry. "These are the habits that mentally strong people rely on" *World Economic Forum.* https://www.weforum.org/agenda/2016/10/habits-to-help-you-develop-mental-strength, October 26, 2016.

246

- Travis Bradberry. "13 Things Mentally Strong People Won't Do". https://www.linkedin.com/pulse/13-things-mentally-strong-people-wont-do-dr-travis-bradberry/, September 11, 2017.

247

- Jeff Haden. *The Motivation Myth.* p. 32. New York: Penguin, 2018.

248

- Travis Bradberry. "These are the habits that mentally strong people rely on" *World Economic Forum.* https://www.weforum.org/agenda/2016/10/habits-to-help-you-develop-mental-strength, October 26, 2016.

249

- Jeff Haden. *The Motivation Myth.* p. 37. New York: Penguin, 2018.

250

- Jeff Haden. *The Motivation Myth.* p. 136. New York: Penguin, 2018.

251

- Travis Bradberry. "13 Things Mentally Strong People Won't Do". https://www.linkedin.com/pulse/13-things-mentally-strong-people-wont-do-dr-travis-bradberry/, September 11, 2017.

252

- Dick Van Dyke. *My Lucky Life*. (New York: Random House, 2011) p. 184.

253

- "Fred Astaire Dancer (1899–1987)" *The Biography.com website*. https://www.biography.com/people/fred-astaire-9190991, Last Updated, April 27, 2017.

254

- Travis Bradberry. "13 Things Mentally Strong People Won't Do". https://www.linkedin.com/pulse/13-things-mentally-strong-people-wont-do-dr-travis-bradberry/, September 11, 2017.

255

- Travis Bradberry. "12 Habits of Genuine People". https://www.linkedin.com/pulse/importance-being-genuine-dr-travis-bradberry/, November 15, 2015.

256

- Travis Bradberry. "Eight Habits of Considerate People". https://www.linkedin.com/pulse/eight-habits-considerate-people-dr-travis-bradberry, November 8, 2017.

257

- *Vincent van Gogh Gallery*. http://www.vggallery.com/, accessed July, 30 2015.
- *Heilbrunn Timeline of Art History*. The Metropolitan Museum of Art. http://www.metmuseum.org/toah/hd/gogh/hd_gogh.htm, accessed July, 30 2015.

258

- Travis Bradberry and Jean Greaves. *Emotional Intelligence 2.0.* p. 188. San Diego, California: TalentSmart, 2009.

259

- Travis Bradberry. "Eight Habits of Considerate People". https://www.linkedin.com/pulse/eight-habits-considerate-people-dr-travis-bradberry, November 8, 2017.

260

- Dan Michel, *Remorse of Conscience*, or *Ayenbite of inwyt*, ed. Richard Morris (London: N. Trubner & Co., 1895) pp. 74-75. Morris' 1895 republication is from Michel's 1340 translation from French to Kentish. Michel's 1340 translation is of the 13th century French *Somme le Roi*. My quote is from a translation of the 1340 Kentish into modern English, translation by Judith G. Humphries, in "The Personification of Death in Middle English Literature" (Denton, Texas: 1970, North Texas State University) p. 10.

261

- Travis Bradberry. "Eight Habits of Considerate People". https://www.linkedin.com/pulse/eight-habits-considerate-people-dr-travis-bradberry, November 8, 2017.

262

- Travis Bradberry. "13 Habits of Exceptionally Likeable People". https://www.linkedin.com/pulse/13-habits-exceptionally-likeable-people-dr-travis-bradberry, January 27, 2015.

263

- Travis Bradberry. "13 Habits of Exceptionally Likeable People". https://www.linkedin.com/pulse/13-habits-exceptionally-likeable-people-dr-travis-bradberry, January 27, 2015.

264

- Travis Bradberry and Jean Greaves. *Emotional Intelligence 2.0.* pp. 160, 161. San Diego, California: TalentSmart, 2009.

265

- Richard Alan Krieger. *Civilization's Quotations: Life's Ideal.* (New York: Algora Publishing, 2002) p. 122.

266

- Benjamin Disraeli, Earl of Beaconsfield, quoted in *Puck*, Volume XV, No. 370 (p. 95). April 9, 1884. Google digitized version: https://books.google.com/books?id=0_kiAQAAMAAJ&pg=PA95.

267

- Aristotle. *Goodreads*.
  http://www.goodreads.com/quotes/31240-happiness-is-a-state-of-activity, July 24, 2015.

268

- Bruno S. Frey, Christine Benesch, Alois Stutzer. "Does watching TV make us happy?" *Journal of Economic Psychology*, Volume 28, Issue 3, June 2007. Elsevier B.V. (ScienceDirect.com).
  http://www.bsfrey.ch/articles/459_07.pdf, February 14, 2007.

269

- Travis Bradberry and Jean Greaves. *Emotional Intelligence 2.0.* p. 124. San Diego, California: TalentSmart, 2009.

270

- Shawn Achor. "The Happy Secret to Better Work" *Ted Talk*. February, 2012.
  https://www.ted.com/talks/shawn_achor_the_happy_secret_to_better_work/transcript?language=en.

271

- Martha Washington. *Letter to Mercy Warren*. 1789.
  https://en.wikiquote.org/wiki/Martha_Washington.

272

- Leslie Becker-Phelps. "Don't Just React: Choose Your Response" *Psychology Today*.
  https://www.psychologytoday.com/blog/making-change/201307/dont-just-react-choose-your-response, July 23, 2013.

273

- Franklin Delano Roosevelt. *AZQuotes*.
  http://www.azquotes.com/quote/250883.

274

- Travis Bradberry and Jean Greaves. *Emotional Intelligence 2.0.* p. 61. San Diego, California: TalentSmart, 2009.

275

- Travis Bradberry. "These are the habits that mentally strong people rely on" *World Economic Forum.* https://www.weforum.org/agenda/2016/10/habits-to-help-you-develop-mental-strength, October 26, 2016.

276

- "Cognitive reflection test" *Wikipedia.* https://en.wikipedia.org/wiki/Cognitive_reflection_test, accessed 12/30/2017.

277

- Marcus Tullius Cicero. *De Oratore,* Book II §36. Paraphrase "Historia magistra vitae est" commonly extrapolated from the quote "Historia vero testis temporum, lux veritatis, vita memoriae, magistra vitae, nuntia vetustatis, qua voce alia, nisi oratoris, immortalitati commendatur" The Loeb Classical Library, English translation Cambridge, Massachusetts, Harvard University Press, 1967. https://archive.org/stream/cicerodeoratore01ciceuoft/cicerodeoratore01ciceuoft_djvu.txt, 55 BC.

278

- Jeff Haden. *The Motivation Myth.* p. 112. New York: Penguin, 2018.

279

- Travis Bradberry and Jean Greaves. *Emotional Intelligence 2.0.* pp. 51, 52. San Diego, California: TalentSmart, 2009.

280

- Travis Bradberry and Jean Greaves. *Emotional Intelligence 2.0.* pp. 7, 8. San Diego, California: TalentSmart, 2009.

- Shawn Achor. "The Happy Secret to Better Work" *Ted Talk*. February, 2012. https://www.ted.com/talks/shawn_achor_the_happy_secret_to_bett er_work/transcript?language=en.

281

- Lisa Quast. "Why Grit Is More Important Than IQ When You're Trying To Become Successful" *Forbes*. https://www.forbes.com/sites/lisaquast/2017/03/06/why-grit-is-more-important-than-iq-when-youre-trying-to-become-successful/, March 6, 2017.

282

- Shawn Achor. "The Happy Secret to Better Work" *Ted Talk*. February, 2012. https://www.ted.com/talks/shawn_achor_the_happy_secret_to_bett er_work/transcript?language=en.

283

- Jon Morrow. "How to Be Smart in a World of Dumb Bloggers" *BoostBlogTraffic*. http://boostblogtraffic.com/smart-blogger/, September 17, 2013.
- Jon Morrow. "On Gluttony, Selfishness, and Unleashing the Power Within" *BoostBlogTraffic*. http://boostblogtraffic.com/unleash-your-power/, November 27, 2014.

284

- Jon Morrow. "How to Be Smart in a World of Dumb Bloggers" *BoostBlogTraffic*. http://boostblogtraffic.com/smart-blogger/, September 17, 2013.

285

- Jeff Haden. *The Motivation Myth*. p. 137. New York: Penguin, 2018.

286

- Belle Beth Cooper. "How to Be a Success at Everything" *Fast Company*. https://www.fastcompany.com/3056613/how-i-became-a-morning-person-read-more-books-and-learned-, February 12, 2016.

287

- Nielsen. "Percentage of Americans who say they watch too much TV: 49 %" *BLS American Time Use Survey*, A.C. Nielsen Co. http://www.statisticbrain.com/television-watching-statistics/, Date Verified: 12.7.2013.
- Robert Kubey and Mihaly Csikszentmihalyi "Television Addiction Is No Mere Metaphor" *Scientific American*. http://www.academia.edu/5065840/Television_Addiction_is_no_mere_metaphor, January 23, 2016.
  Further Information from the authors on television addiction:
  - Television and the Quality of Life: How Viewing Shapes Everyday Experience. Robert Kubey and Mihaly Csikszentmihalyi. Lawrence Erlbaum Associates, 1990.
  - Television Dependence, Diagnosis, and Prevention. Robert W. Kubey in Tuning in to Young Viewers: Social Science Perspectives on Television. Edited by Tannis M. MacBeth. Sage, 1995.
  - "I'm Addicted to Television": The Personality, Imagination, and TV Watching Patterns of Self-Identified TV Addicts. Robert D. McIlwraith in Journal of Broadcasting and Electronic Media, Vol. 42, No. 3, pages 371--386; Summer 1998.
  - The Limited Capacity Model of Mediated Message Processing. Annie Lang in Journal of Communication, Vol. 50, No. 1, pages 46--70; March 2000.
  - Internet Use and Collegiate Academic Performance Decrements: Early Findings. Robert Kubey, Michael J. Lavin and John R. Barrows in Journal of Communication, Vol. 51, No. 2, pages 366--382; June 2001.
- "Television Addiction" *All About Life Challenges*. http://www.allaboutlifechallenges.org/television-addiction.htm, accessed September 21, 2014.

288

- Dick Van Dyke. *My Lucky Life*. (New York: Random House, 2011) pp. 21–22.

289

- Peter Falk. *Just One More Thing*. (New York: Carroll & Graf, 2007) pp. 165–166.

Made in the USA
Columbia, SC
21 May 2018